CLEAN EATING FOR THE SMART

Healthy & Delicious

Recipes to Perfect Health

DIANA WATSON

DEDICATION

I dedicate this book to my two beautiful children and my loving husband who have been nothing short of being my light and joy throughout the years.

throughout the United States.

The information in the following pages is broadly considered to be a truthful and accurate account of facts and as such any inattention, use or misuse of the information in question by the reader will render any resulting actions solely under their purview. There are no scenarios in which the publisher or the original author of this work can be in any fashion deemed liable for any hardship or damages that may befall them after undertaking information described herein.

Additionally, the information in the following pages is intended only for informational purposes and should thus be thought of as universal. As befitting its nature, it is presented without assurance regarding its prolonged validity or interim quality. Trademarks that are mentioned are done without written consent and can in no way be considered an endorsement from the trademark holder

Table of Contents

Part 1

Introduction

Chapter 1: What Clean Eating Is

Chapter 2: Benefits of Clean

Eating

Part 2

Chapter 1: The Keto Plan & How it

Part 3

Chapter 1: Mastering the Air Fryer

VIP Subscriber List

Dear Reader, If you would like to receive latest tips and tricks on cooking, weight-loss, cookbook recipes, upcoming books & promotions, and more, do subscribe to my mailing list in the link below! I will be giving away a free book that you can download right away as well after you subscribe to show my appreciation!

Here's the link: http://bit.do/dianawatson

Introduction

Congratulations on purchasing this book, and making the decision to live a healthier, happier life! *Clean Eating; Healthy & Delicious Recipes to Perfect Health* is the definitive guide on learning what exactly clean eating is, and how to get there to achieve your goals!

The following book will discuss exactly what clean eating is, and what it isn't. Also, included within the pages of this book you will learn:

- What clean eating isn't
- Why clean eating is good for you
- The top 10 most common genetically modified foods

- How your body and waistline will thank you when you decide to eat clean

There are many books about clean eating out there, thank you for choosing this one. Every effort was made to explain the basics, help guide you on where to start, and encourage you to make better choices to take care of YOU!

Chapter 1: What Clean Eating Is

So, you want to get healthy, feel better, maybe lose a few pounds, and you keep hearing about clean eating everywhere, right? Although at a glance, making the decision to clear your kitchen and eat clean may seem daunting, it doesn't have to be! I promise, clean eating is NOT. THAT. HARD. Before we look at what clean eating really means, let's discuss what it isn't. Clean eating is not:

- A diet. This is not a diet, or a quick fix to shed a few pounds.
- A torture mechanism. You are in no way going to be deprived of the food you love.

- A perfect practice. Clean eating is a journey, not a destination. Clean eating isn't an elitist gimmick or fad, it is a lifestyle change.

Now that you can breathe a little easier knowing that nobody is going to judge you, and that clean eating is not reserved for the perfect and always polished, let's talk about what clean eating really is.

Clean eating is about eliminating foods from your diet that aren't really foods at all, getting rid of foods and ingredients that have zero nutritional benefits, and getting back to basics. Food should feed our bodies, minds, and souls. Food should not be made in a laboratory, genetically toyed with, or leave our bodies unsatisfied and unhealthy. Food is fuel, but it should be fuel we share with our loved ones, enjoyed, and above all, good for us!

Let's Get Started

Where does one begin the journey to kicking the junk? Well, that really depends on how far you are willing to take things, and your comfort level. Everyone wants to look and feel better, and clean eating will help you achieve those goals. But, almost everything in your pantry and kitchen is full of stuff you do not need. Below is an idea of where to start cleaning up your diet for the better.

Kick the preservatives, chemicals, and processed food.

I know this seems daunting when you really consider what is on the grocery store shelves today, but you can start small. Chips are great and all, but check out that back label. Can you pronounce all the ingredients and do you know what they are? Are there more than 5 ingredients? Can you thinly slice potatoes and bake or broil them? If you answered no to all the above questions, you may starve. Just kidding! The point here is to really think about what is in those chips, and whether you are ready to either substitute them in your diet, or if it is easier to eliminate them all together. You can eat what you want, but do you really think those bagged chips are fueling your body in a healthy way considering the label?

Eliminate GMO foods wherever you can

And while chips are an easy target, consider the ears of corn at your local grocers. They are big, bright, and look really yummy, but so very bad. Most corn is genetically modified, so check the stickers, take note of the display, or ask an employee. Buying certified organic fresh produce is a great way to ensure that your food is GMO free. Organic does sometimes cost more, but buying seasonal produce from a local market is usually not any costlier than what you can get at major chain grocery stores. And, you are doing your local economy a huge favor. To start small, consider buying organic, and replacing your current selections of the notorious top ten listed below.

The top 10 genetically modified foods are:

- Soy
- Dairy Products
- Corn
- Rice
- Tomatoes
- Potatoes
- Canola
- Papaya

- Peas

The list above is a good place to start. The goal is to get clean, not stress yourself out. There is no shame in starting small and working your way from there. Any positive, healthy changes will have your body thanking you, Trust me.

Chapter 2: Benefits of Clean Eating

So, what are the benefits of eating clean? Consider that you are getting rid of foods that are not only lacking nutritional value, but that these foods also contain a varying array of toxins, poisons, and additives that can make you prone to illnesses that can literally kill you. Clean eating will eliminate the garbage, and fill your body with nutrient rich foods. Foods that are dense in nutrients help your body build and maintain a healthier gut, which in turn translates into a healthier, more effective immune system. You will not only be less likely to get sick, you will also be decreasing your chances of forming chronic illnesses, many of which are linked to the chemicals, preservatives, and GMO's that many people ingest daily.

Another awesome side effect of eating clean is that by eating cleaner, you are eating healthier. Most people that make the change report healthy, steady, weight loss, and that is a bonus for most of us! Eating clean foods chock full of nutrition, you will also feel fuller on less weight per average meal. Imagine a wrap that weighs 6 ounces filling you up better than a frozen pizza that weighs 16 ounces, and gives you more energy. Speaking of energy...

Eating clean will give you more energy, and your energy levels will maintain better throughout the course of the day. By eliminating empty carbohydrates, refined and sugar foods, and steering clear of refined grains, your body will begin regulate its insulin levels naturally. No spike in blood sugar equals no sugar crash later.

Clean eating also encourages an increase in Omega-3 fatty acids in your diet, which help your brain. B complex vitamins are good for your entire system, and increase serotonin and dopamine chemicals released by the brain, making you feel happier. And, Omega-3 fatty acids have been shown to reduce moodiness and even help decrease depression. Another benefit to eating clean is that you will sleep better too! Passing on a cookie and milk before bed and instead noshing on a handful of almonds (which contain tryptophan) and skim milk (that offers us melatonin) will help you sleep like a baby, and wake up refreshed. There are a thousand reasons why clean eating is good for you, and your body will only thank you!

PART 2

Chapter 1: The Keto Plan & How it Works

You will soon understand how you can eat most of the

foods you always enjoy. You will be able to make some substitutes to get going which are described in this chapter.

Happy Discovery!

Several Types of Keto Diet Plans

- *Plan 1*: You can choose from the standard ketogenic diet (SKD) which consists of high-fat, moderate protein, and is extremely low in carbs.

- *Plan 2*: The cyclical ketogenic diet or CKD is created with 5-keto days trailed by two high-carb days.

- *Plan 3*: The targeted keto diet, which is also called TKD, will provide you with a plan to add carbs to the diet during the times when you are working out.

- *Plan 4*: The high-protein ketogenic diet is very similar to the standard keto plan in all aspects except that it has more protein.

However, let's not get too far ahead of the plan. You need to focus on the first 30 days! The long process to explain each of these types would take another entire book!

Health Benefits from a Ketogenic Diet Plan

These are just a few of the ways you can benefit from remaining on the diet plan. It's hard to believe a diet plan can remedy so many health issues.

Acne: Your insulin levels are lowered by consuming less sugar and eating less processed foods. The acne will begin to clear up as you continue with the plan.

Alzheimer's disease: The symptoms and progression will be slowed.

Lowered Blood Pressure: While using the keto plan; you are experiencing reduced intake of carbs which will reduce your blood pressure levels. It is recommended to seek advice from your regular doctor to see if it is possible to reduce some of your medication while you are on the keto diet. You may also have some dizziness when you first begin the plan which is one of the first indications that the plan is working. The result is a lack of carbohydrates.

Cancer: Slow tumor growths and several other types of cancer have shown improvement with the keto plan.

Diabetes and Pre-diabetes: The main link to pre-diabetes is excess body fat which is removed which is proven by research that insulin sensitivity was improved by as much as 70%.

Epilepsy: Children's research studies have proven the diet works in the reduction of seizure activity.

Gum Disease: The sugar you consume influences the pH balance in your mouth. If you have issues before you begin the plan; you should begin to see a remarkable improvement within approximately three months.

Obesity: When the ketogenic diet plan is followed—the weight will dissolve.

Stiffness and Joint Pain: It is important to continue with the elimination of any grain-based foods. It is believed that the grains are one of the largest factors which cause the pain. Just remember "no grain—no pain."

Thinking is Improved: You might be a bit foggy-minded when you first begin the plan since you will be consuming high-fat foods. After all, your brain is about 60% fat by weight; your thinking skills should improve with the intake of the fatty foods indicated with the keto diet.

The Elements of Ketosis

Ketosis is used to help your burn body fat and drop extra pounds. Proteins will fuel your body to burn the fat—therefore—the ketosis will maintain your muscles and make you less hungry.

Your body will remain healthy and work as it should. If you don't consume enough carbs from your food; your cells will begin to burn fat for the necessary energy instead. Your body will switch over to ketosis for its energy source as your cut back on your calories and carbs.

Two elements that occur when your body doesn't need the glucose:

Lipogenesis: If there is a sufficient supply of glycogen in your liver and muscles, any excess is converted to fat and stored.

Glycogenesis: The excess of glucose converts to glycogen and is stored in the muscles and liver. Research indicates that only about half of your energy used daily can be stored as glycogen.

As a result, your body will have no more food—similar to when you are sleeping—your body burns the fat and creates ketones. These ketones break down the fats, which generate fatty acids, and burn-off in the liver through beta-oxidation.

Simply stated, when you no longer have a supply of glycogen or glucose, ketosis begins and will use the consumed/stored fat as energy.

The Internet provides you with a keto calculator to use at http://keto-calculator.ankerl.com/. You can check your levels when you want to know what essentials your body needs during your diet plan or after. All you need to do is document your personal information such as weight and height. The calculator will provide you with the essential math.

Weight Loss and Protein

Protein needs to be in your plan for these reasons:

Protein is a Fat Burner: Science has proven your body cannot use and burn your fat as energy sources unless you have help from either carbs or protein. The balance of protein must be maintained to preserve your calorie-burning lean muscles.

Protein Saves Your Calories: Protein slows down your digestion process making you feel more satisfied from the foods you eat. During the first cycle of your diet plan; it is imperative that you feel full, so there is no temptation to cheat on the strategy.

Muscle Repair and Growth: Protein should be increased on days when you are more active. It is essential to have a plan on what your meals will consist of with a balance of carbs, proteins, and calories. The balance is what you are attempting to achieve with a focused plan such as the keto diet.

The Role of Calories, Protein, and Carbs

Calories are held within your body with the use of the

nutrients of protein, fat, and carbs which your body will use for energy.

Carbohydrates

Your body exchanges one-hundred percent of the carbs into glucose which gives your body an energy boost. About 50% to 60% of your intake of calories is produced by carbs. Carbs stored in your liver as glycogen is released as your body needs it. Glucose is essential for the creation of adenosine triphosphate (ATP) which is an energy molecule. The fuel from glucose is vital for the daily maintenance and activities inside your body. After the liver has reached its maximum capacity for its limits, the excessive carbohydrates turn into fat.

Count Those Carbs

Before you are totally in gear, you need to start carb counting to make sure you keep your body in perfect 'sync' with the plan. Reading the labels may be a bit nerve-racking in the beginning, but after a while, it will be as you have always done it that way.

Remember this Formula: Total Carbs minus (-) Fiber = Net Carbs

A rough estimate will include you consuming between 20 to 30 carbs daily. It is almost a necessity to own a set of food scales to take out the guesswork.

Keep this information in mind before you make the purchase:

- *The Automatic Shut-Off*: Seek a scale that does not have this option. The result could be you being in the midst of a recipe—move the dish—and the scale could reset; NOT.

- *The Tare Function*: When you set a bowl on the scale, the feature will allow you to reset the scale back to zero (0).

- *Removable Plate*: Keep the germs off of the scale by removing the plate. Be sure it will come off to eliminate the bacterial buildup.

- *Seek a Conversion Button*: You need to know how to convert measurements into grams since not all recipes have them listed. The grams keep the system in complete harmony.

Natural Supplements for Ketogenic Dieters

Fermented Foods: Use items, while on the keto plan such

as coconut milk kefir, coconut milk, yogurt, pickles, sauerkraut, and kimchi to help with any digestive issues.

Lemon and Lime: Your blood sugar levels will naturally drop with these citric additions, and signal a boost in your liver function. Use them in green juices, with a salad, or with cooked with meats or veggies. The choices are limitless and assist you with the following:

- Reduces toothache pain
- Boosts your immune system
- Relieves respiratory infections
- Balances pH
- Decreases wrinkles and blemishes
- Reduces fever
- Excellent for weight loss
- Flushes out the unwanted, unhealthy materials
- Blood purifier

Apple Cider Vinegar: Who would believe the benefits you can receive from just one to two tablespoons of vinegar in an 8-ounce glass of water would help the process? You can choose the straight up method and skip the water. These are just a few ways this helps your progress:

- Reduces cholesterol

- Excellent for detoxification

- Helps you to drop the pounds

- Improves your digestion tract

- Helps with sore muscles

- Controls sugar intake/aids in diabetes

- Strengthens your immune system

- A good energy booster

- Balances your inner body system and functions

Cinnamon: Use cinnamon as part of your daily plan to improve your insulin receptor activity. Just put one-half of a teaspoon of cinnamon into a shake or any type of keto dessert. Many of the keto recipes contain the ingredient.

Turmeric: Dating back to Ayurveda and Chinese medicine the is of this Asian orange herb has been known for its anti-inflammatory compounds. Add it to you smoothies, green drinks, meats, or veggies. These are some of its benefits:

- Prevents Alzheimer's disease

- Weight management

- Relieves arthritis

- Reduces your cholesterol levels

- Helps control diabetes

- Improves your digestion

Be Aware of Some Foods and Beverages: Which Ones to Avoid

Agave Nectar: One teaspoon has 5 grams of carbs versus 4 grams in table sugar.

Beans and Legumes: This group to avoid includes peas, lentils, kidney beans, and chickpeas. If you use them, be sure to count the carbs, protein, and fat content.

Cashews and Pistachios: The high carb content should be monitored for these yummy nuts.

Fruits: Raspberries, blueberries, and cranberries contain high sugar contents. In small portions; you can enjoy some strawberries.

Grains and Starches: Avoid wheat-based items such as cereal, rice, or pasta.

Hydrogenated Fats: Cold-pressed items should be avoided when using vegetable oils such as safflower, olive, soybean, or flax. Coronary heart disease has been linked to these fats which also include margarine.

Tomato-based Products: Read the labels because most of the tomato products contain sugar. If you use them be sure to account for the sugar content. (The recipes provided have considered this.)

Chapter 2: The 14-Day Plan

Day One

Breakfast: Keto Scrambled Eggs

Ingredients

3 large eggs

Fresh ground pepper

Coarse salt

1 tablespoon unsalted butter

Instructions

1. Whisk the eggs in a bowl.

2. Use low heat and place the butter into a skillet.

3. Add the eggs. Continue to stir until well-done, usually 1 ½ to 3 minutes.

Serving Portion: Fat: 26.3 g; Carbs 1.8 g; Protein: 17.4 g; Calories: 318

Lunch: Tuna Cheese Melt (Low-Carbs)

Ingredients

2 Pieces of "Oopsie" bread

Ingredients for the Salad

1 to 2 Celery stalks

5 1/3 Tablespoons sour cream or mayonnaise

1 Can tuna (in olive oil)

4 Tablespoons chopped dill pickles

½ teaspoon lemon juice

Pepper and salt to taste

½ minced clove garlic

Toppings

A pinch of paprika powder or cayenne pepper

3 ½ ounces shredded cheese

Serving Ingredients

Olive oil

1/3 Pound leafy greens

"Oopsie" Bread (makes six to 8)

3 Eggs

A pinch of salt

4 ¼ ounces cream cheese

½ teaspoon baking powder

½ Tablespoon ground psyllium husk powder

Instructions

1. Preheat the oven to 350ºF. Put parchment paper onto a cookie sheet.

2. Blend all of the salad ingredients.

3. Place the bread slices on the prepared sheet, spread the tuna, and sprinkle the cheese on top of each slice of bread.

4. Sprinkle some cayenne or paprika powder on the sandwich halves and bake in the oven for about 15 minutes.

5. Have some leafy greens with a drizzle of olive oil.

"Oopsie" Bread Instructions

1. Heat the oven to oven at 300ºF.

2. Begin by separating the egg whites (whites in one bowl and yolks in the other).

3. Whisk the egg whites with the salt until peaks are formed.

4. Combine the cream cheese and egg yolks—add the baking powder and psyllium seed husk (making it more Oopsie type bread).

5. Blend/fold in the whites into the yolk mixture —keeping out the air in the whites of the eggs.

6. Place six or eight 'oopsies' on the paper-lined sheet.

7. Bake on the center oven rack, usually for 25 minutes or until browned.

Dinner: Chicken Smothered in Creamy Onion Sauce

Ingredients

1 whole green/spring onion

2 tablespoons or 1-ounce butter

4 chicken breast halves (skinless—boneless)

8 ounces sour cream

½ teaspoon sea salt

Note: The chicken should weigh approximately six ounces or 170 g for this recipe.

Instructions

1. In a large pan, melt the butter on the stovetop using the med-high setting. Lower the heat setting to med-low—put the chicken with the butter—cover and cook about ten more minutes.

2. Chop the onion using just the white and green sections.

3. Flip the breasts—cover and simmer—another 8 or 9 minutes (or until completely done).

4. Combine the onion, and continue cooking the chicken for another one or two minutes.

5. Take it off of the burner, and blend in the salt and sour cream.

6. Let the meal rest and flavors blend for five minutes.

Stir well and serve.

Day Two

Breakfast: Mock Mc Griddle Casserole

Ingredients

1 pound breakfast sausage

¼ cup flaxseed meal

1 cup almond flour

10 large eggs

6 tablespoons maple syrup

4 ounces cheese

4 tablespoons butter

¼ teaspoon sage

½ teaspoon each: onion & garlic powder

Instructions

1. Heat the oven to 350ºF. Use parchment paper to line a 9 x 9-inch casserole dish.

2. Using medium heat; start cooking the breakfast sausage on the stove in a skillet.

3. Blend all of the dry (the cheese included) ingredients and add the wet ones.

4. Add four tablespoons of the syrup and blend well.

5. After the sausage is crispy brown—blend all of the ingredients; (the fat too).

6. Pour the mixture into the dish and sprinkle the remainder of the syrup on the top.

7. Bake for 45 to 55 minutes. Remove it and let it cool.

Yields: Eight Servings

Time Saving Tip: The casserole should be easy to remove by using the edge of the parchment paper.

Lunch: Brussels Sprouts with Hamburger Gratin

Ingredients

1 Pound Ground beef

1 Pound Brussels Sprouts

½ Pound diced bacon

4 tablespoons sour cream

1/3 Pound shredded cheese

1- ¾ Ounces butter

Pepper and salt to taste

1 tablespoon Italian seasoning

Instructions

1. Cut the Brussels sprouts in half.

2. Preheat the oven to 425ºF/220ºC.

3. Saute the Brussels sprouts and bacon in the butter. Flavor with the sour cream and place in a baking pan/dish.

4. Fry the beef and season with pepper and salt; add the herbs and cheese—sprinkling on top of the base layer.

5. Bake on the center rack of the oven for fifteen minutes.

Serve with a dollop of mayonnaise and a fresh salad.

Yields: Four Servings

Dinner: Squash and Sausage Casserole

Ingredients

1 pound browned sausage

2 large eggs

1 medium zucchini (sliced & cooked)

2 medium summer squash (sliced & cooked)

1 teaspoon salt

½ teaspoon onion powder or ¼ cup dried minced onion

1 cup mayonnaise

1 package sugar substitute (or stevia)

¼ teaspoon pepper

1 ½ cups shredded cheddar cheese (divided)

¼ melted butter

Instructions

1. Preset the oven to 350ºF.

2. Blend each of the ingredients except for one-half of a cup of shredded cheese.

3. Put the ingredients into a lightly greased oblong baking plate.

4. Sprinkle the remainder of cheese on the casserole.

5. Bake until lightly browned for approximately thirty minutes.

This casserole will easily serve 12 people with an amazing flavor you won't soon forget!

Day Three

Breakfast: Can't Beat it Porridge

Ingredients

1 cups almond or coconut milk

1 pinch salt

1 Tablespoon each:

- Sunflower seeds

- Chia Seeds

Instructions

1. Using a small saucepan on the stovetop, blend each of the components, and bring to a boiling. Lower the burner and cook slowly until the porridge is the consistency you desire

2. Garnish with some butter or milk. You can also add some fresh unsweetened berries or cinnamon.

Yields: One Serving

Time-Saving Tip: Make it ahead of time using a big glass jar. Fill the jar with the following ingredients and shake them up. Each serving will correspond with three tablespoons for each serving.

These are the ingredients needed for the batch:

1 Tbsp. cinnamon

½ tsp. salt

1 1/4 cup each:

- Sunflower seeds

- Flaxseeds

- Chia seeds

Lunch: Salad From a Jar

Ingredients

1 (4-ounce) rotisserie chicken/smoked salmon/other protein

1 ounce each:

- Cucumber

- Cherry tomatoes

- Leafy greens

- Bell pepper

4 tablespoons olive oil or mayonnaise

½ Scallion

Instructions

1. Chop or shred the veggies and place the leafy greens to the bottom for a crunch followed by the colorful veggies. (You can also use some cauliflower or broccoli for a change of pace.)

2. Top it off with some of the grilled protein of your choice. You can also use cold cuts, tuna fish, mackerel or boiled eggs.

3. Cheese cubes, seeds, nuts, and olives are also healthy and colorful additions.

4. Add a generous amount of mayonnaise or salad dressing and enjoy!

Yields: One Serving

Dinner: Ham and Cheese Stromboli

Ingredients

1 large egg

1 ¼ cups shredded mozzarella cheese

3 tablespoons coconut flour

4 tablespoons almond flour

4 ounces of ham

1 teaspoon Italian seasoning

3 ½ ounces cheddar cheese

Instructions

1. Preheat the oven to 400ºF.

2. Melt the mozzarella cheese in the microwave for one minute/alternating at ten-second intervals; stirring until melted.

3. In a mixing bowl, blend the coconut and almond flour with the seasonings.

4. Toss in the mozzarella on the top and work it in.

5. After the cheese has cooled; beat the egg and combine everything

6. On a flat surface; put some parchment paper, and add the mixture.

7. Use a rolling pin or your hands to flatten the mix.

8. Place several diagonal lines using a knife or pizza cutter. (Leave a row of approximately four inches wide in the center.

9. Alternate the layers using the cheddar and ham on the uncut space of dough until you have used all of the fillings.

10. Bake for 15 to 20minutes or it is browned.

Day Four

Breakfast: Frittata with Cheese and Tomatoes

Ingredients

6 eggs

2/3 cup soft cheese (ex. Feta 3 ½ ounces or 100 g)

½ medium white onion (1.9 ounces or 55 g)

2/3 cup halved cherry tomatoes

2 tablespoons chopped herbs (ex. basil or chives)

1 tablespoon ghee/butter

Instructions

1. Heat the oven broiler to 400°F.

2. Place the onions on a greased, hot iron skillet, and cook with ghee/butter until slightly brown.

3. In a separate container, crack the eggs and add the salt, pepper, or add herbs of your choice. Whisk and add to the onion pan.

4. Cook until the edges begin to get brown. Top with the cheese and tomatoes.

5. Put the pan in the broiler for five to seven minutes or until done.

Lunch: Chicken—Broccoli—Zucchini Boats

For a variety textures as well as flavors to spice up lunch; this is the one!

Ingredients

6 ounces shredded chicken

2 tablespoons butter

2 hollowed-out zucchini (10 ounces)

3 ounces shredded cheddar cheese

1 stalk of green onion

1 cup broccoli

2 tablespoons sour cream

Instructions

1. Heat the oven temperature to 400ºF.

2. Slice the zucchini lengthwise and scoop most of
    the insides out until you have a shell of
    approximately ½ to 1 cm. thick.

3. Melt one tablespoon of the butter into each boat,
    flavor with a dash of pepper and salt, and bake
    them for around twenty minutes.

4. Shred the chicken, cut the broccoli florets into
    small pieces, and Measure out six ounces of
    cheese. Blend in with the sour cream.

5. Remove the zucchini shells when done and add the
    mixture.

6. Sprinkle each of them with the remainder of the
    cheese.

7. Bake for another ten or fifteen minutes until the
    cheese is browned and melted.

8. Use a bit of sour cream, mayonnaise, or chopped
    onion as a garnish.

Dinner: Steak-Lovers Slow-Cooked Chili

Ingredients for Chili:

1 cup beef or chicken stock

½ cup sliced leeks

2 ½ pounds (1-inch cubes) steak

2 cups whole tomatoes (canned with juices)

1 tablespoon chili powder

½ tsp. salt

1/8 tsp. ground black pepper

¼ tsp. ground cayenne pepper

½ tsp. cumin

Optional Toppings

1 teaspoon fresh chopped cilantro

2 tablespoons sour cream

¼ cup shredded cheddar cheese

½ avocado (cubed or sliced)

Instructions

1. Place all of the items except the topping fixings into the slow cooker.
2. Set the cooker on the high setting for about six hours.

Yields: Twelve Servings

Serving Portion: 1: Fat: 26.0 g; Carbs 3.3 g; Protein: 38.4 g; Calories: 321

Servings with Toppings: *Serving Portion: 1:* Fat: 41.32 g; Carbs 13.49 g; Protein: 32.47 g; Calories: 540.33

Day 5

Breakfast: Brownie Muffins

Ingredients

½ tsp. salt

1 cup flaxseed meal

¼ cup cocoa powder

½ Tbsp. baking powder

1 Tbsp. cinnamon

2 Tbsp. coconut oil

1 large egg

1 tsp. vanilla extract

¼ cup sugar-free caramel syrup

½ cup pumpkin puree

¼ cup slivered almonds

1 tsp. apple cider vinegar

Instructions

1. Heat the oven temperature at 350ºF.

2. In a deep mixing bowl—combine all of the ingredients—mixing well.

3. Use six paper liners in the muffin tin, and add ¼ cup of the batter to each one.

4. Sprinkle several almonds on the tops, pressing gently.

5. Bake approximately fifteen minutes. It is done when the top is set.

Serving Portion: 1 muffin (The recipe serves six): Fat: 13.4 g; Carbs 8.2 g; Protein: 7 g; Calories: 183.3

Lunch: Bacon-Avocado-Goat Cheese Salad

Ingredients

½ Pound bacon

½ Pound goat cheese

4 ounces walnuts

2 avocados

4 ounces arugula lettuce

Ingredients for the Dressing

7 ½ tablespoons mayonnaise

Juice of ½ of a lemon

2 tablespoons heavy whipping cream

7 ½ tablespoons olive oil

Instructions

1. Preheat the oven temperature to 400ºF/200ºC.

2. Prepare a baking dish with some parchment paper.

3. Slice the goat cheese into ½-inch round slices and put in the baking dish. Place on the upper rack of the oven.

4. Pan-fry the bacon until crunchy.

5. Cut the avocados and place on top of a bed of lettuce, add the bacon, cheese, and nuts to the top of your creation.

6. Make the dressing using a stick blender. Sprinkle in a dash of pepper, salt, or a few fresh herbs.

Yields: Four Servings

Dinner: Tenderloin Stuffed Keto Style

Ingredients

2 pounds pork tenderloin or venison

½ cup feta cheese

½ cup gorgonzola cheese

1 teaspoon chopped onion

2 tablespoons crushed almonds

2 garlic cloves, minced

½ teaspoon each: fresh ground black pepper and sea salt

Instructions

1. Preheat the grill.

2. Form a pocket in the tenderloin.

3. Mix the cheeses, almonds, garlic, and onions.

4. Stuff the pocket, and seal using a skewer.

5. Grill until its desired doneness.

Yields: Eight Servings

Serving Portion: 1: Fat: 6.2 g; Carbs 2.9 g; Protein: 28.8 g; Calories: 194

Day 6

Breakfast: Sausage—Feta—Spinach Omelet

Ingredients

½ tablespoon extra-virgin olive oil

2 sausage links

3 large eggs

¼ cup Half & Half

1 cup spinach

1 tablespoon feta cheese

Note: You will need two skillets for this yummy omelet!

Instructions

1. Use medium heat for both pans, and pour olive oil in one of the two.

2. In a small dish, use the Half & Half and mix with the eggs—add the seasonings—and scramble.

3. In the clean pan, cook the sausage.

4. Sauté the spinach in the oiled pan—add a pinch of salt and pepper if desired.

5. After both have finished cooking; put them together in a bowl.

6. Transfer the olive oiled pan to the sausage fat pan —and add the eggs.

7. When the edges begin to cook—add the spinach, sausage, and cheese. Cook another minute—flip the omelet. Cook another two to three minutes.

8. Cover one pan with the other and let the combo steam.

9. Remove and enjoy your masterpiece!

Serving Portion: Fat: 43 g; Carbs 3 g; Protein: 31 g; Calories: 535

Lunch: Pancakes with Cream-Cheese Topping

Don't be alarmed, this is an excellent choice for any time and is so healthy.

Ingredients

8 ¾ ounces cottage cheese

5 eggs

1 tablespoon ground psyllium husk powder

A pinch of salt

For Frying: Coconut oil or butter

Ingredients for the Topping

2 tablespoons red or green pesto

½ pound (8 ounces) ricotta or cream cheese

2 tablespoons olive oil

Ground black pepper and Sea Salt

½ thinly sliced red onion

Instructions

1. Combine one tablespoon of the olive oil with the pesto and cream cheese; set aside.

2. Using a hand blender, mix the salt, cottage cheese, eggs, and husk powder; blend until smooth. Let rest for ten minutes.

3. On the stovetop using the medium heat setting; heat two tablespoons of the oil or butter.

4. Drop several dollops of the cheese batter (2 to 3 inches in diameter), frying the pancakes a few minutes per side.

5. Serve with a few red onion slices with a drizzle of oil, pepper, and salt. You can also use fresh herbs, smoked fish roe or chopped chives.

Dinner: Skillet Style Sausage and Cabbage Melt

Ingredients

4 spicy Italian chicken sausages

2 tablespoons coconut oil

½ cup diced onion

1 ½ cups purple cabbage

1 ½ cups green cabbage

2 tablespoons chopped fresh cilantro

2-1-ounce slices Colby jack cheese

Instructions

1. Start by removing the sausage casings and rough-chopping them. Shred the cabbage and chop the onions.

2. Add the coconut oil, cabbage, and onion in a large skillet using the med-high setting for approximately eight minutes (the veggies should be tender).

3. Blend the cheese and cover.

4. Turn the heat off and let it rest five minutes as the cheese melts.

5. When it is time to serve—stir gently and add the cilantro.

Yields: Four Servings

Serving Portion: 1: Fat: 14.62 g; Carbs 3.52 g; Protein: 18.26 g; Calories: 231

Day 7

Breakfast: Tapas

Have a great mixture!

Ingredients

Cold Cuts:

- Prosciutto

- Serrano ham

- Salami

- Chorizo

Cheeses:

- Gouda

- Parmesan

- Mozzarella

- Cheddar

Veggies:

- Pickled cucumbers

- Peppers

- Radishes

- Cucumbers

Avocado with pepper and homemade mayonnaise

Fresh Basil

Splash of freshly squeezed lemon juice

Nuts:

- Hazelnuts

- Almonds

- Walnuts

Instructions

1. Cut all of the ingredients into cubes or sticks and split the avocado cutting its fruit into small wedges.

2. Blend with four ounces of mayonnaise pepper and maybe a splash of lemon juice

3. Use the avocado shells for the serving platter.

Yields: Four Servings

Lunch: Tofu—Bok-Choy Salad

Tofu Ingredients:

15 ounces extra firm tofu

2 teaspoons minced garlic

Juice from ½ a lemon

1 tablespoon each:

- sesame oil

- water

- soy sauce

- rice wine vinegar

Bok Choy Salad Ingredients:

2 tablespoons soy sauce

1 stalk green onion

2 tablespoons chopped cilantro

9 ounces bok choy

3 tablespoons coconut oil

1 tablespoon Sambal Olek

Juice of ½ of a lime

1 tablespoon peanut butter

7 drops liquid Stevia

Instructions

1. Press the tofu in towels for approximately five to six hours to dry.

2. Combine each of the marinade ingredients.

3. When dry; chop the tofu into squares and put in a plastic container/bag with the marinade sauce.

4. Leave it to sit for at least thirty minutes—preferably overnight.

5. Heat the oven to 350ºF. Bake for 30 to 35 minutes on a parchment paper-lined baking dish or a Silpat (non-stick baking sheet with a blend of fiberglass mesh and silicone).

6. In the interim, combine the dressing ingredients (except for the bok choy) in a mixing dish. Toss in the onion and cilantro.

7. Chop the bok choy as you would cabbage, into small slices.

8. Remove the tofu—combine, and enjoy.

Note: Bok choy is a Chinese vegetable.

Serving Portion: Fat: 35 g; Carbs 7.3 g; Protein: 25.0 g;

Calories: 442.3

Dinner: Hamburger Stroganoff

Ingredients

8 ounces sliced mushrooms

1 pound ground beef

2 minced cloves of garlic

2 Tbsp. butter

1 ¼ cups sour cream

1/3 cup water or dry white wine

1 tsp. lemon juice

¼ tsp. paprika

1 tsp. dried parsley

Substitute: You may also use one tablespoon fresh chopped parsley.

Instructions

1. Sauté the onions and garlic in a skillet prepared using one tablespoon of butter.

2. Mix in the beef into the pan— sprinkle with pepper and salt if desired. Cook until done and set to the side.

3. Use the remainder of the butter, the mushrooms, and the wine/water, and add them to the pan. Cook until half of the liquid is reduced and the mushrooms are soft.

4. Take them off the burner—add the paprika and sour cream.

5. On low heat stir in the meat and lemon juice.

Use additional spices for flavoring if desired.

Serving Portion: 1 (272 g): Fat: 28.1 g; Carbs 6.1 g; Protein: 38.7 g; Calories: 447

Day 8

Breakfast: Cheddar—Jalapeno Waffles

Ingredients

3 large eggs

1 small jalapeno

3 ounces cream cheese

1 tablespoon coconut flour

1-ounce cheddar cheese

1 teaspoon each:

- baking powder
- Psyllium husk powder

Instructions

1. Combine all of the ingredients using an immersion blender (except for the jalapeno and cheese) until it has a smooth texture.

2. Add the cheese and jalapeno; blend and pour into the waffle iron.

3. You can garnish with your favorite ingredients in about five or six minutes total

Note: Psyllium husk is a native of Pakistan, Bangladesh, and India. It is available online at several locations

Serving Portion: 2 waffles: Fat: 28 g; Carbs 6 g; Protein: 16 g; Calories: 338

Lunch: Salmon Tandoori with Cucumber Sauce

Ingredients

1 ½ Pounds Salmon (In pieces)

2 tablespoons coconut oil

1 tablespoon tandoori seasoning

Ingredients for the Cucumber Sauce

½ cup shredded cucumber

1 ¼ cup sour cream or mayonnaise

2 minced garlic cloves

Juice of ½ of a lime

Optional: ½ teaspoon salt

Ingredients for the Crispy Salad

3 ½ ounces arugula lettuce

3 scallions

1 yellow pepper

Juice of 1 lime

2 avocados

Instructions

1. Preheat the oven to 350ºF.

2. Mix the tandoori seasoning and the 2 tablespoons of oil to coat the salmon.

3. Bake the salmon for fifteen to twenty minutes.

4. Combine the lime juice, garlic, cucumber (blot the water out with paper towels first), and sour cream/mayonnaise in a mixing dish.

5. Prepare the salad ingredients and enjoy.

Yields: Four Servings

Dinner: Ground Beef Stir Fry

Ingredients

300 g (approximately 10 ½ ounces) ground beef

5 medium brown mushrooms

½ cup broccoli

2 leaves kale

½ medium Spanish onion

1 Tbsp. coconut oil

½ medium red pepper

1 Tbsp. cayenne pepper

1 Tbsp. Chinese Five Spices

Note: McCormick was used for the Five Spices

Instructions

1. Prepare the vegetables—slice the mushrooms—chop the broccoli.

2. Heat a frying pan on the stovetop using the med-high setting. Pour in the oil and toss in the onions. Cook for an additional minute.

3. Blend the remainder of the vegetables and cook an additional two minutes—stirring often.

4. Combine the spices and beef—lower the heat to medium—and continue cooking for approximately two more minutes.

5. Cover the pan and cook for five or ten more minutes until the beef is done.

Serving Portion: 1 (Recipe is for three servings): Fat: 18 g; Carbs 7 g; Protein: 29 g; Calories: 307

Day 9

Breakfast: Cheddar and Sage Waffles

Ingredients

1 1/3 coconut flour

1 teaspoon ground sage

½ teaspoon salt

¼ teaspoon garlic powder

3 teaspoons baking powder

2 cups canned coconut milk

½ cup water

3 tablespoons melted coconut oil

1 cup shredded cheddar cheese

2 eggs

Instructions

1. Prepare the waffle iron on the required manufacturer's setting. Grease the iron (top and bottom).

2. Blend all of the seasonings, flour, and baking powder in a container.

3. Mix the wet ingredients, stirring until the batter becomes stiff. Blend in the cheese.

4. Scoop out a one-third cup of the batter and place in each section of the iron.

5. Depending on how you like your waffles; you can run them through two cycles on the iron if you want it crispier.

Serving Portion: 1 waffles (The recipe serves 12): Fat: 17.21 g; Carbs 9.2 g; Protein: 6.52 g; Calories: 213.97

Lunch: Crispy Shrimp Salad on an Egg Wrap

Ingredients for the Wraps

1-ounce butter

4 eggs

Pepper and salt to taste

Shrimp Salad Ingredients

6 ounces shrimp

2 avocados

1/2 of an apple/handful of radishes

1 teaspoon lime juice

1 celery stalk

1 cup mayonnaise

1 red chili pepper

8 tablespoons fresh parsley or cilantro

Instructions for the Wrap

1. Cook and peel the shrimp. Finely chop the red chili pepper and fresh cilantro/parsley.

2. Whip the eggs with the pepper and salt.

3. Using a medium frying pan, melt the butter. Empty half of the egg batter until the egg gets firm, and repeat for the second one.

Instructions for the Salad

1. Slice the avocado and scoop out providing you with ½-inch cubes. Place them in a dish and

give a fresh squeeze of juice over them and mix.

2. Dice the apple and thinly slice the celery, putting them with the avocado. Blend in the peppers, cilantro/parsley, and mayonnaise.

3. Combine well and gently stir in the shrimps. Add more salt if desired.

Yields: Two Servings

This is one of those meals that can be enjoyed with leafy greens or alone. Add a couple of boiled eggs in place of the wrap for another healthy choice.

Dinner: Bacon Wrapped Meatloaf

Ingredients

1 finely chopped yellow onion

1 ½ Pounds ground lamb, poultry, pork *or* beef

2 tablespoons butter

8 tablespoons heavy whipping cream

1 egg

6 ¾ tablespoons shredded cheese

1 tablespoon dried basil/oregano

1 tsp. salt

½ tsp. black pepper

7 ¾ ounces sliced bacon

Optional: ½ tablespoon tamari soy sauce

For the Gravy: 1 ¼ cups heavy whipping cream

Instructions

1. Preheat the oven to 400ºF/200ºC.

2. Saute the onion in a pan with the butter, but don't brown it.

3. Combine the meat in a container, adding all of the remainders of ingredients but omit the bacon. Don't over-work it, but blend the ingredients well, making a loaf.

4. Bake it in the center of the oven for approximately 45 minutes. You can use some aluminum foil to cover the meatloaf, just in case, the bacon begins to scorch.

5. Reserve any of the accumulated juices and make the gravy, blending it with the cream in a small saucepan.

6. Let the mixture come to a boil using low heat until it is creamy and the right texture, usually for approximately ten to fifteen minutes.

7. Spice it up with a drizzle of tamari soy sauce for a bit of flavor.

8. Have some cauliflower or broccoli on the side with some butter. It is all up to you to decide on the veggie choices.

Yields: Four Servings

Day 10

Breakfast: Omelet Wrap with Avocado & Salmon

Ingredients

3 large eggs

½ package smoked salmon (100 g or 1.8 ounces)

½ avocado (3.5 ounces or 100 g)

1 spring onion (1/2 ounce or 15 g)

2 tablespoons cream cheese (full-fat—2.3 ounces or 64 g)

2 tablespoons chives (freshly chopped)

1 tablespoon butter or ghee

Instructions

1. In a mixing bowl—add a pinch of pepper and salt along with the eggs. Use a fork or whisk—mixing them well. Blend the chives and cream cheese.

2. Prepare the salmon and avocado (peel and slice).

3. In a sauté pan, melt the butter/ghee, and add the egg mixture. Cook until fluffy.

4. Put the omelet on a serving dish, and spoon the mixture of cheese over it.

5. Sprinkle the onion, prepared avocado, and salmon into the wrap.

Close and enjoy!

Serving Portion: Fat: 66.9g; Carbs 13.3 g; Protein: 36.9 g

Lunch: Tuna Avocado Melt

Ingredients

1-10 - ounce can drained tuna

1 medium cubed avocado

¼ cup mayonnaise

1/3 cup almond flour

¼ teaspoon onion powder

¼ cup parmesan cheese

½ teaspoon garlic powder

1/2 cup coconut oil (for frying)

Instructions

1. In a mixing container, blend all of the ingredients except for the coconut oil and avocado. Fold the cubed avocado into the tuna.

2. Make balls and coat each one with the almond flour.

3. Use the medium heat setting and put the oil in a pan—mix the tuna—and continue cooking until brown.

Note: Some people like to use this as a casserole dish.

Yields: Twelve Servings

Per Serving Portion: Fat: 11.8 g; Carbs 2.0 g; Protein: 6.2 g; Calories: 134.7

Dinner: Hamburger Patties with Fried Cabbage

Ingredients for the Hamburger Patties

1 egg

1 ½ Pounds ground beef

3 ¼ ounces feta cheese

1 tsp. salt

¼ tsp. ground black pepper

1 ¾ ounces finely- chopped, fresh parsley

1-ounce butter

1 tablespoon olive oil

Ingredients for the Gravy

1 ¾ - Ounces fresh (coarsely chopped) parsley

1 ¼ cups heavy whipping cream

Pepper and Salt

2 tablespoons tomato paste

Ingredients for the Green Cabbage

4 ¼ ounces butter

1 ½ Pounds shredded green cabbage

Pepper and Salt

Instructions

1. Form eight oblong patties by blending all of the ingredients listed under the hamburger patties.

2. Using the med-high setting on the stovetop, prepare a skillet with olive oil and butter and fry the patties for a minimum of ten minutes.

3. Empty the whipping cream and tomato paste into the mixture—stir—and let them blend.

Serve with some parsley for garnishment.

Instructions for Butter-fried Green Cabbage

1. Use a food processor or knife to shred the cabbage.

2. Prepare a frying pan with the butter and sauté the cabbage for approximately fifteen minutes on the med-high setting.

3. Reduce the heat for the last five minutes (or so)—stirring regularly.

Variations: You can also enjoy this with whatever you desire, including spinach, carrots, mushrooms, acorn squash, or corn.

Yields: Four Servings

Day 11

Breakfast: The Breadless Breakfast Sandwich

Ingredients

4 Eggs

1-ounce ham/pastrami cold cuts

2 tablespoons butter

2 ounces of Adam/provolone/cheddar cheese

Several drops of Worcestershire or Tabasco sauce

Pepper and salt to taste

Instructions

1. Cut the cheese into thick slices.

2. Prepare a frying pan over medium heat. Fry the eggs over-easy with a pinch of pepper and salt.

3. Add the choice of meat onto the two eggs, a layer of cheese, and the egg for the top of the 'bun.'

4. Give the sandwich a splash of Worcestershire sauce/Tabasco and serve. You can also use some French Dijon mustard to complement the ham.

Yields: Two Servings

Lunch: Thai Fish With Coconut & Curry

Ingredients

1 ½ Pounds whitefish/salmon

4 tablespoons butter/ghee

Pepper and salt

1 to 2 tablespoons green/red curry paste

8 tablespoons fresh chopped cilantro

1 can coconut cream

1 Pound broccoli/cauliflower

For Greasing the Dish: Olive oil/butter

Instructions

1. Grease a baking dish. Preheat the oven to 400ºF.

2. Place the salmon/fish in a dish where there is not any extra space between the dish and fish (not meant as a rhyme).

3. Place a dab of butter on each piece along with a shake of pepper and salt.

4. Combine the chopped cilantro, curry paste and coconut cream in a small container. Pour it over the fish.

5. Bake until the fish is falling apart done, usually about twenty minutes.

6. Boil the broccoli/cauliflower in water (lightly salted) for several minutes as a side dish.

Yields: Four Servings

Dinner: Keto Tacos or Nachos

Ingredients

500 g or 17.6 ounces ground beef

1 medium white onion (3.0 ounces)

4 tacos

1 teaspoon chili powder

2 garlic cloves

½ teaspoon ground cumin

2 teaspoons extra-virgin coconut oil or ghee

1 tablespoon unsweetened tomato puree

1 cup water (8 ounces)

½ teaspoon salt—more or less

Cayenne pepper or freshly ground black pepper

Topping Ingredients

1 small head of lettuce (approximately 3.5 ounces or 100 g)

1 cup or 5.3 ounces cherry tomatoes

1 medium avocado (7.1 ounces or 200 g)

Optional Toppings

4 tablespoons sour cream

1 cup grated cheese

Veggies including cabbage, cucumbers, or peppers

Instructions

1. Using med-high, add some butter/ghee in a frying pan; toss in the onion. Sauté until brown and mix in the beef, continue cooking until the beef is done.

2. Add the cumin and chili powder. (You can substitute with 1 ½ teaspoon of paprika.)

3. Pour in the water and add the tomato puree. Also add pepper, and salt if you like for additional flavoring.

4. Continue cooking until the meat is done and approximately ¼ of the sauce is reduced. Set to the side and prepare the vegetable topping.

5. Use the meat mixture to stuff the shells. Garnish with some of the tomatoes, lettuce, and avocado.

6. As an option, you can add a bit of sour cream or cheddar cheese.

Note: You may use this as a tasty taco or on the side with the meat as the centerfold for the remainder of the veggies.

The choice is all yours!

Day 12

Breakfast: Scrambled Eggs With Halloumi Cheese

Ingredients

5 to 6 eggs

3 ½ ounces diced Halloumi cheese

4 ½ ounces diced bacon

8 tablespoons each:

- Pitted olives

- Chopped fresh parsley

Pepper and Salt to taste

2 scallions

2 tablespoons olive oil

Instructions

1. Dice the bacon and cheese.

2. Over the stovetop, use the medium-high setting; pour the oil into a frying pan. Add the

scallions, cheese, and bacon—sauté until browned.

3. Whip/Whisk the eggs, pepper, salt, and parsley in a mixing container.

4. Pour the mixture into the pan over the cheese and bacon.

5. Reduce the heat—toss in the olives and sauté for several minutes.

6. All Ready! You can enjoy this with or without a salad.

Yields: Two Servings

Lunch: Salmon with Spinach and Chili Tones

Ingredients

1 tablespoon chili paste

1 ½ Pounds Salmon (in pieces)

1 cup sour cream/mayonnaise

1 ¾ cup olive oil/butter

1 Pound fresh spinach

4 tablespoons grated parmesan cheese

Pepper and Salt

Instructions

1. Place the oven setting to 400ºF/200ºC. Use some cooking oil to coat a baking dish/pan.

2. Flavor the salmon with the pepper and salt. Place in the dish skin side down.

3. Blend the chili paste, sour cream/mayonnaise, and parmesan cheese and spread it on the filets.

4. Bake until the salmon is done—usually fifteen to twenty minutes.

5. In the meantime, sauté the spinach until it wilts using the oil/butter.

Yields: Four Servings

Dinner: Chicken Stuffed Avocado—Cajun Style

Ingredients

1 ½ cups cooked chicken (7.4 ounces or 210 g)

2 medium or 1 large avocados (10.6 ounces or 300 g)

2 tablespoons cream cheese/sour cream

2 tablespoons lemon juice (fresh)

¼ cup mayonnaise

½ teaspoon each: onion powder & garlic powder

¼ teaspoon each: salt and cayenne pepper

1 teaspoon each: paprika and dried thyme

Instructions

1. Shred the chicken into small pieces.

2. Blend all of the ingredients—saving the salt and lemon juice until last.

3. Leave one-half to one-inch of the avocado flesh—scoop the middle. Remove the seeds.

4. Cut the center/scooped pieces of avocado into small pieces and fill each of the halves with the mixture of chicken.

Yields: Two Servings

Serving Portion: Fat: 50.6 g; Carbs 16.4 g; Protein: 34.5 g

Day 13

Breakfast: Western Omelet

Ingredients

2 tablespoons sour cream/heavy whipping cream

6 eggs

Pepper and Salt

2 ounces butter

3 ½ ounces shredded cheese

5 ounces of ham

½ each:

- Finely chopped green bell peppers
- Finely chopped yellow onion

Instructions

1. Whisk the sour cream/cream and eggs until fluffy. Flavor with the pepper and salt. Add half of the cheese and combine.

2. Melt the butter on the stovetop on the medium heat setting. Sauté the peppers, onions, and ham for just a few minutes.

3. Pour the batter in and fry until the omelet is almost firm.

4. Lower the heat and Sprinkle the remainder of the cheese on top of your masterpiece. Fold the omelet right away.

Have a fresh green salad as a perfect brunch touch!

Yields: Two Servings

Lunch: Tortilla Ground Beef Salsa

Ingredients

1 ½ Pounds ground lamb/beef

8 to 12 low-carb tortilla breads

2 tablespoons olive oil

1 cup of water

Tex-Mex seasoning (see below)

 1 teaspoon salt

Shredded leafy greens

17 to 27 tablespoons shredded cheese

Salsa Ingredients

1 to 2 diced tomatoes

2 avocados

1 tablespoon olive oil

Juice of 1 lime

8 tablespoons fresh cilantro

Pepper and Salt

Tex-Mex Seasoning

2 tsp. each:

- Paprika powder

- Chili powder

1 to 2 tsp. garlic/onion powder

1 tsp. ground cumin

A pinch of cayenne pepper

Optional: 1 tsp. salt

Instructions

1. Prepare two batches of low-carb tortilla bread (see below).

2. Chop the cilantro. Take out the beef so it can become room temperature. Cold meats can have an effect on the cooking times, and it is more of a boil, not a fry.

3. On the stovetop, heat the oil using a large pan. Toss in the beef, and cook for around ten minutes.

4. Add the salt, water, and taco seasoning to the beef and simmer until most of the liquid has evaporated.

5. Meanwhile, prepare the salsa with all of the ingredients.

6. Serve on the tortilla bread with some shredded cheese along with the leafy greens.

Yields: Four Servings

Low-Carb Tortillas

Ingredients

2 egg whites

2 eggs

6 ounces cream cheese

1 tablespoon coconut flour

1 to 2 teaspoons ground psyllium husk powder

½ teaspoon salt

Instructions

1. Heat the oven to 400ºF. Prepare two baking sheets with parchment paper.

2. Whip the eggs and whites until fluffy. Blend in the cream cheese and whisk until creamy.

3. Combine the coconut flour, psyllium powder, and salt in a small container. Add the flour mixture for the batter a spoon at a time.

4. Spread out the batter on the baking tins, spreading thin, about ¼-inch thick. You can make two rectangles or four to six circles.

5. Bake until the tortilla begins to brown around the edges, usually about five minutes (or so).

6. Serve with some of your *Tex-Mex Ground Beef and Salsa*.

Yields: Two Servings

Dinner: Fish Casserole with Mushrooms

Ingredients

1 Pound mushrooms

3 ¼ ounces butter

2 Tbsp. fresh parsley

1 t. salt

Pepper (to taste)

2 C. heavy whipping cream

2 tablespoons fresh parsley

2 to 3 Tbsp. Dijon mustard

1 ½ Pounds white fish (Ex. Cod)

½ Pound shredded cheese

1 1/3 pounds cauliflower/broccoli

3 ¼ ounces olive oil/butter

Instructions

1. Heat the oven to 350ºF. Lightly grease a baking dish for the fish.

2. Slice the mushrooms into wedges. *Sauté* in a pan with the butter, pepper, salt, and other herbs.

3. Empty the mustard and cream into the mixture and reduce the heat. Simmer for five to ten minutes until the sauce thickens.

4. Flavor the fish with the pepper and salt and add it to the prepared container. Sprinkle with ¾ of the cheese. Pour the creamed mushroom mixture over it and the rest of the cheese as a topping.

5. Bake approximately thirty minutes if the fish are frozen (less if not). After 20 minutes, test the fish to see if it flakes apart easily.

Remember, the fish will cook for several minutes after it is removed from the oven.

6. Prepare the cauliflower into small florets, removing the leaves and stalks. You can use the entire broccoli by cutting it into rods/lengthwise.

7. Boil the veggie of choice, drain and add some butter/olive oil.

8. Coarsely mash with a fork or wooden spoon; adding some pepper and salt, and serve with your fish.

Yields: Four Servings

Day 14

Breakfast: Blueberry Smoothie

Smoothie Ingredients

1 C. fresh or frozen blueberries

1 2/3 C. coconut milk

1 Tbsp. lemon juice

½ tsp. vanilla extract

Instructions

1. Put all of the ingredients into a tall beaker. Mix using a hand mixer.

2. Pour the lemon juice in for additional flavoring.

Notes: You can substitute 1 ¼ cups of Greek yogurt for a dairy option and adjust with a small amount of water if you are searching for more liquid consistency. Add 1 tablespoon of a healthy oil such as coconut for more satiety.

Yields: Two Servings

Lunch: Cheeseburger

Ingredients

7 ounces shredded cheese

1 ½ Pounds ground beef

2 teaspoons each:

- Onion powder

- Garlic powder

- Paprika

For Frying

2 tablespoons fresh oregano

Finely chopped butter

Salsa

2 scallions

2 tomatoes

1 avocado

Fresh Cilantro (to taste)

Salt

1 tablespoon olive oil

Toppings

- Lettuce

- Cooked bacon

- Dijon mustard

- Mayonnaise

- Pickled jalapenos

- Dill pickle

Instructions

1. Chop all of the salsa ingredients in a small container and set to the side.

2. Combine all of the seasonings and ½ of the cheese into the beef mixture.

3. Prepare four burgers and grill or pan fry to your liking—adding cheese at the end of the cooking cycle.

4. Serve on the bed of lettuce with some mustard and a dill pickle.

Yields: Four Servings

Dinner: Turkey with Cream Cheese Sauce

Ingredients

1 1/3 Pounds turkey breast

2 tablespoons butter

2 cups heavy whipping cream/sour cream

7 ounces cream cheese

Pepper and salt

1 tablespoon tamari soy sauce

6 ¾ tablespoons small capers

Instructions

1. Heat the oven to 350ºF.

2. *Sprinkle the turkey with pepper and salt for seasoning.*

3. *Add the butter to a frying pan. Sauté the turkey until golden. Place in the oven to finish cooking.*

4. *Using a small pan, combine the heavy cream/sour cream and cream cheese, bringing it to a boil; lower the heat and cook slowly for a few minutes.*

5. *On high heat in a small pan, use a small amount of butter or oil to fry the capers or enjoy them fresh.*

6. *When the turkey breast and veggies are done, add the sauce and capers on top of the turkey and serve along with some side dishes such as cauliflower or broccoli.*

Yields: Four Servings

Chapter 3: Additional Breakfast Recipes

Chia Pudding

Ingredients

1 cup light coconut milk

¼ cup chia seeds

½ tablespoon light corn syrup

Instructions

1. Combine all of the ingredients in a small mason jar or bowl.

2. Refrigerate overnight. It is ready when the seeds have gelled, and the pudding is thick.

3. Add some nuts and fresh fruit and 'dive in.'

Cow-time Breakfast Skillet

Ingredients

2 medium diced sweet potatoes

1 Pound breakfast sausage

5 eggs

Handful of cilantro

1 diced avocado

Hot sauce

Optional: Raw cheese

Pepper and Salt

Instructions

1. Heat the oven to 400ºF.

2. Use medium heat on the stovetop; place an iron or oven-safe skillet. Crumble and brown the sausage. Remove the sausage, cook the potatoes until crunchy, and reserve the grease.

3. Put the sausage back in the pan. Make some spaces in the 'wells' of the skillet, enough room for one egg. Crack the eggs into each of the wells.

4. Put the skillet into the preheated oven and bake enough for the eggs to set (about 5 minutes). Turn up the thermostat in the oven

to the broil setting to let it broil the tops of the yolks with the crispy sweet potatoes.

5. Take the skillet out of the oven and cover it with some cilantro, avocado, and hot sauce.

Enjoy the different flavors.

Cream Cheese Pancakes

Ingredients for the Pancakes

2 oz. (room temperature) cream cheese

2 organic eggs

½ teaspoon cinnamon

1 teaspoon granulated sugar substitute

Instructions

1. Place each of the pancake ingredients into a blender. Blend until creamy smooth; letting it rest for two minutes for the bubbles to settle back down.

2. Grease a pan with Pam spray or butter.

3. Pour about ¼ of the pancake batter into the hot pan; cook for two minutes. Flip and continue cooking about one more minute.

4. Serve with berries or a sugar-free syrup of your choice.

Yields: Four Pancakes

Serving Size: 1 Batch: Carbs 2.5 g net; Fat 29; Protein 17 g; Calories 344

Dairy-Free Latte

Ingredients

2 Tbsp. coconut oil

1 2/3 C. hot water

2 eggs

1 tsp. ground ginger/pumpkin pie spice

Splash of vanilla extract

Instructions

1. Use a stick blender to combine all of the ingredients.

2. If you want to replace the spices; you can use 1 tablespoon of instant coffee or cocoa.

Enjoy for a quick boost!

Yields: Two Servings

Keto Sausage Patties

Ingredients

1 teaspoon maple extract

2 tablespoons granular Swerve Sweetener

½ teaspoon pepper

1 pound ground pork

2 tablespoons sage (chopped fresh)

1/8 teaspoon cayenne

1 teaspoon salt

¼ teaspoon garlic powder

Instructions

1. Combine each of the ingredients in a large mixing container.
2. Shape the patties to about a one-inch thickness.
3. The recipe will make eight equal patties.
4. Add a small amount of olive oil or a dab of butter to a pan over medium heat. For each side, allow three to four minutes.

Serving Portion: 2 patties: Carbs 1.4 g; Fat: 11 g;

Protein: 21 g; Calories: 187

Keto Bacon

Use the Regular Oven

1. Preheat to 350 ºF.

2. Put the bacon on a baking tray. Bake 20 to 25 minutes

3. Drain on a paper towel.

Use the Microwave

1. Put the bacon on paper towels in a single layer on a microwave-safe dish.

2. Use the high setting for four to six minutes.

Use the Skillet

1. Prepare the pan on the medium-low to medium.

2. Put the bacon into the pan single-layered.

3. Cook until the desired doneness is acquired.

Serving Portion: 2 slices: Fat: 19 g; Carbs 0.0 g; Protein: 7 g; Calories: 200

Mushroom Omelet

Ingredients

3 eggs

7/8 ounces shredded cheese

2 to 3 mushrooms

Optional: 1/5 of an onion

Pepper and salt to taste

For frying: 7/8 ounces butter

Instructions

1. Whisk the eggs with the pepper and salt, add the spices.

2. On the stovetop, use a frying pan to melt the butter. Pour in the eggs.

3. When the omelet begins to cook to firmness; sprinkle the mushrooms, cheese, and onion on top.

4. Ease the edges up using a spatula, and fold in half. Remove from the pan when golden brown.

If you are having brunch; add a crispy salad.

Yields: One serving

Chapter 4: Additional Lunch and Dinner Recipes

Deviled Eggs

With this tasty combination; it is hard to say breakfast or lunch; maybe brunch!

Ingredients

6 large eggs

¼ teaspoon yellow mustard

1 tablespoon mayonnaise

1 teaspoon paprika

Garnish: Parsley/salt/pepper

Optional

- ½ teaspoon cayenne pepper
- Several drops hot sauce
- 1 teaspoon cumin

Instructions

1. Slice the eggs lengthwise.

2. Mix the egg yolks with the rest of the ingredients.

3. Put the goodies inside the egg bed.

4. Sprinkle with condiments as desired.

Serving Portion: Fat: 20 g; Carbs 1 g; Protein: 19 g; Calories: 265

Ham and Apple Flatbread

Crust Ingredients

¾ cup almond flour

2 cups grated mozzarella cheese (part-skim)

2 tablespoons cream cheese

1/8 teaspoon dried thyme

½ teaspoon sea salt

Topping Ingredients

4 ounces sliced ham (low-carb)

½ small red onion

1 cup grated Mexican cheese

¼ medium apple

1/8 teaspoon dried thyme

Instructions

1. Remove the seeds and core from the apples. You can leave them unpeeled but will need to use a vegetable peeler to make the thin slices.

2. Heat the oven to 425ºF.

3. Cut two pieces of parchment paper to fit into a 12-inch pizza pan (approximately two inches larger than the pan).

4. Use the high-heat setting and place a double boiler (water in the bottom pan), and bring the water to boiling. Lower the heat setting and add the cream cheese, mozzarella cheese, salt, thyme, and almond flour to the top of the double boiler—stirring constantly.

5. When the cheese mixture resembles dough, place it on one of the pieces of parchment—and knead the dough until totally mixed.

6. Roll the dough into a ball—placing it at the center of the paper—place the second piece of paper over the top, and roll with a rolling pin (or a large glass).

7. Place the dough onto the pizza pan (leaving the paper connected).

8. Poke several holes in the dough and put into the preheated oven for approximately six to eight minutes.

9. When browned, remove it, and lower the setting of the oven to 350ºF.

10. Arrange the cheese, apple slices, onion slices, and ham pieces.

11. Top off with the remainder (3/4 cup) of cheese.

12. Season with the ground pepper, salt, and thyme.

13. Place the finished product into the oven, baking until you see a golden brown crust.

14. Slide it off the parchment paper and cool two or three minutes before cutting.

Yields: Eight Slices

Tip: If you do not own a double boiler; you can substitute with a mixing dish over a pot of boiling water as a substitute.

Serving Portion: 1: Fat: 20 g; Carbs 5 g; Protein: 16 g; Calories: 255

Chicken Breast with Herb Butter

Ingredients for the Fried Chicken

4 Chicken Breasts

Pepper and Salt

1-ounce of olive oil/butter

Herb Butter Ingredients

1 clove garlic

1/3 Pound Butter (room temperature)

1 tsp. lemon juice

½ tsp. each:

- garlic powder

- salt

4 Tbsp. fresh chopped parsley

Leafy Greens

½ Pound leafy greens (baby spinach for example)

Instructions

1. Take the butter out of the refrigerator for at least thirty to sixty minutes before you begin to prepare your meal.

2. Add all of the ingredients, including the butter, and blend thoroughly in a small container; set to the side.

3. Use the pepper and salt to flavor the chicken. Cook the chicken filets in a skillet using the butter over medium heat. To avoid dried out filets, lower the temperature the last few minutes.

4. Serve over a bed of greens with some melted herb butter over the top.

Yields: Four Servings

Low-Carbonara

Ingredients

2/3 Pounds diced Pancetta/bacon

1 ¼ cups heavy whipping cream

1 tablespoon butter

3 1/3 tablespoons mayonnaise

Fresh chopped parsley

Pepper and salt

2 Pounds Zucchini

3 ½ ounces grated Parmesan cheese

4 egg yolks

Instructions

1. Empty the heavy cream into a saucepan, bringing it to a boil. Lower the burner and continue boiling until the juices are reduced by about a third.

2. Fry the bacon/pancetta; reserve the fat.

3. Combine the heavy cream, mayonnaise, pepper, and salt into the saucepan mixture.

4. Make 'zoodles' out of the zucchini using a potato peeler or spiralizer.

5. Add the zoodles to the warm sauce and serve with egg yolks, bacon, parsley, and freshly grated cheese.

6. Drizzle a bit of the bacon grease on top.

Yummy!

Yields: Four Servings

Pesto Chicken Casserole with Olives and Cheese

Ingredients

1 ½ Pounds chicken breasts/thighs

3 ½ ounces green or red pesto

8 tablespoons pitted olives

1 2/3 cups heavy whipping cream

½ Pound diced feta cheese

Pepper and Salt

1 finely chopped garlic clove

For Frying: Butter

For Serving

- Olive oil

- 1/3 Pound leafy greens

- Sea salt

Instructions

1. Heat the oven to 400ºF.

2. Cut the chicken into pieces and flavor with the pepper and salt.

3. Place in a skillet with the butter, cooking until well done.

4. Combine the heavy cream and pesto.

5. Put the chicken pieces in the baking dish with the garlic, feta cheese, and olives, along with the pesto mix.

6. Bake for 20 to 30 minutes until the perfect color.

Enjoy with some green beans, sautéed asparagus, or another veggie of your choice.

Yields: Four Servings

Red Pesto Pork Chops

Ingredients

4 Pork chops

4 tablespoons red pesto

2 tablespoons olive oil/butter

6 tablespoons mayonnaise

Instructions

1. Thoroughly rub the chops with the pesto.

2. Fry on medium heat in a skillet with oil/butter for eight minutes. Reduce the heat and simmer four more minutes.

3. Serve with the pesto mayonnaise: 6 tablespoons of mayonnaise (+) 1 to 2 tablespoons pesto.

Serve with a large salad. You can also add a serving of cauliflower and broccoli with cheese.

Chapter 5:

Snacks and Desserts for the Diet Plan

Keto Ginger Snap Cookies

Ingredients

¼ cup unsalted butter

1 large egg

2 C. almond flour

½ tsp. ground cinnamon

1 tsp. vanilla extract

1 C. sugar substitute/Erythritol (Swerve)

2 tsp. ground ginger

¼ tsp. each:

- Salt
- Ground cloves
- Nutmeg

Instructions

1. Set the oven to 350ºF.

2. Combine the dry ingredients in a small dish.

3. Combine the remainder components to the dry mixture, and mix using a hand blender/mixer. (The dough will be crumbly and stiff.)

4. Measure out the dough for each cookie and flatten with a fork or your fingers.

5. Bake for approximately nine to eleven minutes or till they are browned.

Yields: 24 Cookies

Pumpkin Pudding

Ingredients

¼ cup pumpkin puree

1/3 cup granulated (Erythritol/Stevia)

½ tsp. pumpkin pie spices

1 tsp. xanthan gum

3 medium egg yolks

1 ½ cups whipping cream

1 tsp. vanilla extract

For the Cream Mixture

3 Tbsp. granulated stevia

1 cup whipping cream

½ tsp. vanilla extract

Instructions

1. Blend the pumpkin spice, xanthan gum, sweetener, and salt. Whip/whisk until the texture is smooth. Add the yolks, puree, and vanilla extract to the mixture; blend thoroughly.
2. Slowly pour in the whipping cream, after all of the cream is added. Using medium heat let the mixture come to a boil.

3. Continue the process for about 4 to 7 minutes, until thickened.

4. Place in the refrigerator in a container. Stir every ten minutes.

5. Meanwhile, in a medium dish, use a mixer to whip the one cup of whipping cream resulting in stiff peaks. Add the vanilla and sweetener; stir gently.

6. After the base pudding mixture has cooled; fold the whipped cream into the mix.

Scoop the pudding into small serving dishes and chill for a minimum of one to two hours.

Note: The Xanthan gum is available on Amazon.

Yields: Six Servings

No-Bake Cashew Coconut Bars

Ingredients

¼ cup maple syrup/sugar-free

1 cup almond flour

¼ cup melted butter

1 teaspoon cinnamon

½ cup cashews

A pinch of salt

1/4 cup shredded coconut

Instructions

1. Combine the flour and melted butter in a large mixing dish.

2. Add the maple syrup, cinnamon, salt, and coconut —blend well.

3. Use roasted or raw cashews. Chop them and add to the cashew-coconut bar dough. Blend well again.

4. Cover a cookie pan with parchment paper and spread the dough onto the paper in an even layer.

5. Place in the fridge for a minimum of two hours. Slice them and enjoy!

Yields: Eight Servings

Brownie Cheesecake

The Brownie Base Ingredients:

2 ounces chopped unsweetened chocolate

2 large eggs

½ cup butter

1/2 cup almond flour

1 pinch of salt

¼ cup cocoa powder

¾ cup granulated Erythritol/Swerve Sweetener

¼ cup pecans/walnuts (chopped)

¼ teaspoon vanilla

Cheesecake Filling Ingredients

2 large eggs

1 pound softened cream cheese

½ cup granulated sugar/Swerve sweetener

½ teaspoon vanilla extract

¼ cup heavy cream

Instructions

1. Butter a nine-inch springform pan; wrapping the bottom with foil.

2. Set the oven at 325ºF.

3. Melt the chocolate and butter in a microwave-safe dish for 30 seconds.

4. Whisk the cocoa powder, almond flour, and salt in a small dish.

5. In a separate dish; whip the vanilla, eggs, and Swerve until smooth.

6. Blend the flour mixture and chocolate/butter mixture. Blend in the nuts.

7. Spread out in the prepared dish and bake for approximately 15 to 20 minutes.

8. Let it cool for about 20 to 25 minutes.

For the Filling

1. Reduce the oven setting to 300ºF.

2. Blend the Swerve, the vanilla, cream, eggs, and cream cheese in a mixing container until everything is thoroughly mixed. Empty the filling ingredients into the crust and place it on a large cookie sheet.

3. Bake for about 35 to 45 minutes. The center should barely jiggle.

4. Loosen the edges with a knife.

5. Place them in the fridge for a minimum of three hours.

Yields: Ten Servings

Chocolate Soufflé

Ingredients

1/3 cup sugar substitute (Lakanto Mont Fruit/Amazon)

1 tablespoon butter

6 large egg whites

3 large egg yolks

5 ounces unsweetened chocolate

Note: The eggs work best at room temperature.

Instructions

1. Preset the oven to 375ºF.

2. Use the butter to grease a soufflé dish.

3. Use a double boiler or a metal dish above a pan of boiling water to melt the chocolate. (Stir the mix constantly.)

4. Remove the dish and whip in the yolks until the mix hardens. Set it to the side.

5. Use a pinch of salt, whip/whisk the egg whites with an electric mixer on the highest setting.

6. Gradually, blend in the sugar/Lakanto. Continue until you see stiff peaks.

7. Stir in one cup of the egg whites into the chocolate combination folding gently using a silicone spatula. Pour the mixture into the soufflé dish.

8. Bake approximately twenty minutes. The center should still jiggle with the soufflé crusted and puffed on the top.

Serve this delicious treat right away.

Topping/Optional: Coconut whipped cream

Yields: Four Treats

Note: To make the soufflé rise evenly; use your thumb to remove the batter from the top of the dish.

Macaroon Keto Bombs

Your curiosity is wondering, "What is a bomb?" The reasoning is that this is good for you and is too delicious to pass by when you are craving a treat!

Ingredients

½ cup shredded coconut

¼ cup almond flour

2 tablespoons sugar substitute (Swerve)

3 egg whites

1 tablespoon each:

- Coconut oil

- Vanilla extract

Instructions

1. Set the oven at 400ºF.

2. In a small container, combine the almond flour, coconut, and Swerve.

3. Use a small saucepan to melt the coconut oil. Add the vanilla extract.

4. *Note*: To mount the egg whites, place a medium dish in the freezer.

5. Add the oil to the flour mixture and blend well.

6. Break the egg whites in the cold dish and whip until stiff peaks are formed. Blend the egg whites into the flour mixture.

7. Spoon the mixture into a muffin cup or place them on a baking sheet.

8. Bake the macaroons for eight minutes or until you see browned edges.

9. Cool the bombs before you attempt to remove them from the pan.

Yields: Ten Servings

Index for Recipes

Chapter 2: The 14-Day Plan

Day One

- Breakfast: Keto Scrambled Eggs

- Lunch: Tuna Cheese Melt (Low-Carbs)

- "Oopsie" Bread

- Dinner: Chicken Smothered in Creamy Onion
  Sauce

Day Two

- Breakfast: Mock Mc Griddle Casserole

- Brussels Sprouts with Hamburger Gratin

- Dinner: Squash and Sausage Casserole

Day Three

- Breakfast: Can't Beat it Porridge

- Lunch: Salad From a Jar

- Dinner: Ham and Cheese Stromboli

Day Four

- Breakfast: Frittata with Cheese and Tomatoes

- Lunch: Chicken—Broccoli—Zucchini Boats

- Dinner: Steak-Lovers Slow-Cooked Chili

Day 5

- Breakfast: Brownie Muffins

- Lunch: Bacon-Avocado-Goat Cheese Salad

- Dinner: Tenderloin Stuffed Keto Style

Day 6

- Breakfast: Sausage—Feta—Spinach Omelet

- Lunch: Pancakes with Cream-Cheese Topping

- Dinner: Skillet Style Sausage and Cabbage Melt

Day 7

- Breakfast: Tapas

- Lunch: Tofu—Bok-Choy Salad

- Dinner: Hamburger Stroganoff

Day 8

- Breakfast: Cheddar—Jalapeno Waffles

- Lunch: Salmon Tandoori with Cucumber Sauce

- Dinner: Ground Beef Stir Fry

Day 9

- Breakfast: Cheddar and Sage Waffles

- Lunch: Crispy Shrimp Salad on an Egg Wrap

- Dinner: Bacon Wrapped Meatloaf

Day 10

- Breakfast: Omelet Wrap with Avocado & Salmon

- Lunch: Tuna Avocado Melt

- Dinner: Hamburger Patties with Fried Cabbage

Day 11

- Breakfast: The Breadless Breakfast Sandwich

- Lunch: Thai Fish With Coconut & Curry

- Dinner: Keto Tacos or Nachos

Day 12

- Breakfast: Scrambled Eggs With Halloumi Cheese

- Lunch: Salmon with Spinach and Chili Tones

- Dinner: Chicken Stuffed Avocado—Cajun Style

Day 13

- Breakfast: Western Omelet

- Lunch: Tortilla Ground Beef Salsa

- Low-Carb Tortillas

- Dinner: Fish Casserole with Mushrooms

Day 14

- Breakfast: Blueberry Smoothie

- Lunch: Cheeseburger

- Dinner: Turkey with Cream Cheese Sauce

Chapter 3: Additional Breakfast Recipes

- Chia Pudding

- Cow-time Breakfast Skillet

- Cream Cheese Pancakes

- Dairy Free Latte

- Keto Sausage Patties

- Keto Bacon

- Mushroom Omelet

Chapter 4: Additional Lunch and Dinner Recipes

- Deviled Eggs

- Ham and Apple Flatbread

- Chicken Breast with Herb Butter

- Low-Carbonara

- Pesto Chicken Casserole with Olives and Cheese

- Red Pesto Pork Chops

Chapter 5: Snacks and Desserts for the Diet Plan

- Keto Ginger Snap Cookies

- Pumpkin Pudding

- No-Bake Cashew Coconut Bars

- Brownie Cheesecake

- Chocolate Soufflé

Macaroon Keto Bombs

PART 3

Chapter 1: Mastering the Air Fryer

How to Use the Air Fryer

The Air Fryer provides you with a way to eat healthier by providing you healthier ways to prepare your recipes without losing the texture and flavor of your homemade meals and snacks. From *French toast sticks* to *air fried ravioli* or that plateful of *Mozzarella sticks* you have been

122

craving; you will enjoy every morsel as you learn how to prepare the recipes provided in this book.

Useful Guidelines for Recipe Measurement

With so many recipes in circulation for the air fryer (AF) provided greatly due to the Internet; you may begin to notice the many different ways they are written. This is because they travel worldwide and the best ones become viral.

These are some of the conversion tables that will guide you through the process:

Celsius to Fahrenheit

Grams to Cups

Grams to Pounds

Milliliters to Cups

Other abbreviations can include the following:

- Cup = C.

- Tablespoon = Tbsp. = T.

- Teaspoon = tsp. = t.

Going by the 'rule-of-thumb,' a handful should be between 1/3 cup to a ½ cup (more or less). You might also hear a smidge or a pinch which is usually a ¼ teaspoon or a dollop is usually a heaping tablespoon.

Tips for Using the Air Fryer

Tip #1: Many pre-made packaged food items you already purchased can be cooked using the Air Fryer. Each food may vary with its cooking time. As a guideline, reduce the cooking times by about 70% compared to times in a conventional oven.

Tip #2: While cooking smaller items such as fries or wings; you can make sure they are cooking evenly by shaking the basket several times during the cooking process.

Tip #3: It is important to pat food items dry if you have marinated or soaked them in to help eliminate splattering or excessive smoke.

Tip #4: It is tempting when you are in a rush to attempt to overload the Air fryer. Don't put too much in the cooking basket at one time. You won't receive the best results if the air cannot make the 360º turns that make the cooker so unique.

Tip #5: Allow at least three minutes warm-up time each time you use the fryer so it can reach its correct starting temperature.

Tip #6: When it comes time to clean the cooking basket, loosen any food particles remaining attached to the basket. Soak each of the attachments in a soapy water solution before scrubbing or placing it in the dishwasher.

Tip #7: If you use aluminum foil or parchment paper, leave a one-half-inch space around the bottom edge of the basket.

Tip #8: Cooking sprays are an excellent choice to spray on your food before cooking. You can also spray the mesh of the cooking basket to keep anything from sticking to its surface.

Proof You Should Own an Air Fryer

Benefit #1: It is a beginner's treat. You can locate your favorite recipes and whip up a remarkable meal at home in half of the time. The machine does the hard work for you. All you need to do is program the temperature and times.

Benefit #2: The Fryer Needs Less Oil: It won't be necessary to add oil to the cooker if you have frozen products which are meant for baking. You only need to adjust the timer and cook. All of the excess fat will drip away into a tray beneath the basket.

You can cook whatever meats you enjoy and receive delicious and healthy results. You will understand this once you begin trying out some of these new recipes. For example; you can cook French fries with a tablespoon of oil versus a vat of oil.

Benefit #3: No Oily Clean Up: You only need to remove the cooking bowl, drip pan, or the cooking basket. It is inside a cover which means you won't have oil vapor deposits on the walls, floors, or countertops.

You can use the dishwasher to clean the movable parts. You can also use a sponge to clean the bits of food that might be stuck to the AF surfaces.

Benefit #4: Purchase Less Oil: It is possible to splurge on the more expensive oils since you only use such a minimal amount.

Benefit #5: Multitasking Features: The Air Fryer is capable of functioning as so many products, whether you need an oven, a hot grill, a toaster, a skillet, or a deep fryer—it is your answer! It can be used for breakfast, lunch, dinner, desserts, and even snacks.

Benefit #6: Safety Functions: The machine will automatically shut down when the cooking time is completed. You will have less burned or overheated food items.

The unit will not slip because of the non-slip feet which help eliminate the risk of the machine from falling off of the countertop. The closed cooking system helps prevent burns from hot oil or other foods.

Now that you know how to avoid some of the pitfalls you may have with your new Air Fryer unit; you can begin planning which delicious treat you want to test first!

Chapter 2: Air Fryer Breakfast Recipes

Apple Dumplings

Ingredients

2 Tbsp. raisins

2 small apples (peeled—cored)

1 Tbsp. brown sugar

2 sheets puff pastry

2 Tbsp. melted butter

Instructions

1) Preheat the Air Fryer to 356ºF.

2) Mix the sugar and raisins.

3) Place each apple on one of the pastry sheets and fill with the raisins/sugar.

4) Fold the pastry over until the apple and raisins are fully covered.

5) Place them on a piece of foil so they cannot fall through the fryer.

6) Thoroughly brush them with the melted butter.

7) Set the timer for 25 minutes. It is ready when the apples are sold and browned.

Note: Be sure to use very small apples for this yummy treat.

Banana Fritters

Ingredients

8 ripe peeled bananas

3 Tbsp. corn flour

One egg white

3 Tbsp. vegetable oil

¾ cup breadcrumbs

Instructions

1) Preheat the fryer at 356ºF.

2) In a skillet using the low heat setting; pour the oil and toss in the breadcrumbs, cooking until golden brown.

3) Use the flour to coat the bananas; dip them into the egg white, and coat them with the breadcrumbs.

4) Place the bananas on a single layer of the basket and air fry for eight minutes.

5) Remove and sit on paper towels.

What a delicious treat to be served warm!

Tip: If you have too many breadcrumbs; you can place them in the fridge in an airtight container to use sometime in the future.

French Toast Sticks

Ingredients

2 gently beaten eggs

4 slices of desired bread

2 tablespoons soft margarine or butter

Cinnamon

Salt

Ground cloves

Nutmeg

Garnish: Maple syrup

Instructions

1) Preheat the Air Fryer to 356ºF.

2) Whisk the eggs, a shake of nutmeg, cloves, and cinnamon together in a small bowl.

3) Spread butter on both sides of the bread, and cut them into strips.

4) Dredge each of the reductions in the egg mix, and arrange in the fryer. (You will need to make two batches.)

5) Pause the fryer after two minutes, remove the pan, and spray the bread with cooking spray.

6) Flip and spray the other side, returning them to the AF for an additional four minutes, making sure they do not burn.

7) It's ready when it is golden brown; serve them immediately.

Garnish with some maple syrup or whipped cream.

Yields: Two Servings

Bacon and Eggs

Ingredients

4 eggs

12 (1/2-inch thick) slices of bacon

Pepper and salt

1 Tablespoon butter

2 sliced croissants

4 Tablespoons softened butter

BBQ Sauce Ingredients

1 C. ketchup

¼ C. apple cider vinegar

2 Tablespoons each:

- Brown sugar

- Molasses

½ teaspoon each:

- Onion powder

- Mustard powder

1 Tablespoon Worcestershire sauce

½ teaspoon liquid smoke

Instructions

1) Preset the temperature in the Air Fryer to 390ºF.

2) On the stovetop, using medium heat—mix the molasses, ketchup, brown sugar, vinegar, onion powder, and mustard powder using a small saucepot. Whisk the liquid smoke and Worcestershire sauce into the mixture to blend thoroughly. Cook until the sauce thickens. Add additional flavoring as desired.

3) Place the bacon on the trays and cook for five minutes. Remove and brush the bacon with the barbecue sauce –flip—and brush the other side —return to the cooker and continue cooking another five minutes.

4) Butter the halved croissant and toast it in the fryer.

5) In the meantime, use a non-stick pan using the med-low setting on the stovetop—melt the butter. Add four eggs to the pan, cooking until the white starts setting—flip and cook about thirty more seconds.

6) Remove from the pan, and enjoy with the bacon and croissant.

Yields: Four Servings

Cheesy Mushroom, Ham, and Egg

Ingredients

3 slices honey shaved ham

1 croissant

4 halved cherry tomatoes

4 small quartered button mushrooms

1 egg

1.8 ounces mozzarella or cheddar cheese

Optional: ½ roughly chopped rosemary sprig

Instructions

1) Lightly grease a baking dish with butter to prevent the mixture from sticking.

2) Preset the Air Fryer to 320ºF.

3) Place the ingredients on 2 layers of cheese in the center and top layer.

4) Make a space in the center of the ham and crack the egg.

5) Sprinkle the rosemary and a smidgen of salt and pepper for flavoring over the mixture.

6) Put it into the preheated basket for eight minutes. Take the croissant out of the AF after four minutes to allow more time for the egg to cook.

Yields: One Serving

Scrambled Eggs

Ingredients

2 eggs

Pepper and salt to taste

Instructions

1) Preset the Air Fryer to 284ºF for about five minutes.

2) Put the butter in the fryer to melt, and spread it out evenly.

3) Empty the eggs and any other ingredients such as cheese or tomatoes.

4) Open the AF every few minutes to whisk to the desired yellow and fluffy consistency.

Make a scrambled egg sandwich or with toast on the side.

Air Fryer Spinach Frittata

For a fantastic meal good for breakfast, lunch, dinnertime, or anytime; you have found it!

Ingredients

1/3 package (or so) of spinach

1 small minced red onion

Mozzarella cheese

3 eggs

Instructions

1) Preset the Air Fryer at 356ºF for at least three minutes.

2) Add oil to a baking pan for one minute.

3) Add the onions and continue cooking for two to three minutes; toss in the spinach and cook three to five minutes additional minutes.

4) Whisk in the eggs, add the seasonings, cheese, and add to the pan.

5) Cook for eight minutes. Season with salt and pepper.

Bacon Wrapped Tater Tots

Ingredients

3 tablespoons sour cream

1 pound sliced bacon (medium)

1 large bag crispy tater tots

4 scallions

½ cup shredded cheddar cheese

Instructions

1) Preheat the Air Fryer to 400ºF.

2) Wrap each of the tots in bacon and place them into the fryer basket. Don't overcrowd, keep them in a single layer.

3) Set the AF timer for 8 minutes.

4) When the timer beeps; place the tots on a plate.

5) Serve with the scallions and cheese garnish. Add a dash of sour cream and enjoy.

Yields: Four Servings

Buttermilk Biscuits

These have to be considered for breakfast also because they are so delicious!

Ingredients

½ C. cake flour

¾ tsp. salt

1-¼ C. all-purpose flour

¼ tsp. baking soda

1 teaspoon granulated sugar

½ tsp. baking powder

¾ C. buttermilk

4 Tbsp. unsalted cold butter (cut into cubes) + melt 1 Tbsp.

Optional for Serving:

Honey or preserves

Butter

Note: Additional flour is needed for dusting the counter or cutting board.

Instructions

1) Preheat the Air Fryer to 400ºF.
1) Sift together the all-purpose flour, sugar, cake flour, baking soda, and the salt in a medium mixing dish.
2) Use a pastry cutter (or your fingers) to blend the ingredients into pea-sized consistency. Pour in the buttermilk and stir using a rubber spatula (or your hands), and make a dough ball. Try not to over-mix the dough.

3) Sprinkle some flour on the counter surface and begin to press the dough into about a ½-inch thickness. It should be approximately eight inches in diameter.

4) Use a cutter to cut the dough into biscuits; dip the tip of the tip of the cutter with the flour making a swift cut. If you twist the dough; it could prevent it from rising.

5) Place the biscuits in a pan and brush them with the melted butter. Place the dough in the basket of the fryer and set the timer for eight minutes.

Enjoy the finished product with some honey or your favorite preserves, jam, or jelly.

Vegan Mini Bacon Wrapped Burritos

Ingredients

2 servings Tofu Scramble or Vegan Egg

2-3 tablespoons tamari

2 tablespoons cashew butter

1-2 tablespoons water

1-2 tablespoons liquid smoke

4 pieces of rice paper

Vegetable Add-Ins

8 strips roasted red pepper

1/3 cup sweet potato roasted cubes

1 small sautéed tree broccoli

Handful of greens (kale, spinach, etc.)

6-8 stalks of fresh asparagus

Instructions

1) Line the pan used for baking with parchment. Preheat the Air Fryer to 350ºF.

2) Whisk the tamari, cashew butter, water, and liquid smoke; set to the side.

3) Prepare the fillings.

4) Hold a rice paper under cool running water— getting both sides wet—just a second. Place on the plate to fill.

5) Start by filling the ingredients –just-off- from the center—leaving the sides of the paper free.

6) Fold in two of the sides as you would when you make a burrito. Seal them and dip each one in the liquid smoke mixture—coating completely.

7) Cook until crispy; usually about eight to ten minutes.

Yields: Four Mini Burritos

Chapter 3: Lunch Recipes

Grilled Cheese Sandwich

Ingredients

½ Cup sharp cheddar cheese

4 Slices white bread or brioche

¼ Cup melted butter

Instructions

1) Pre-set the Air Fryer temperature to 360ºF.

2) Spread butter on each side of all of the bread slices, and put the cheese on two of them; putting them together. Cook until browned, about five to seven minutes.

Yields: Serves Two

Cheeseburger Mini Sliders

Ingredients

6 Slices cheddar cheese

1 Pound ground beef

6 Dinner Rolls

Black pepper and Salt

Instructions

1) Pre-set the heat on the Air Fryer to 390ºF.

2) Form 6 (2 ½-ounce) patties and flavor with the pepper and salt

3) Place the burgers on the AF basket for ten minutes.

4) Take them from the cooker and add the cheese; returning to the Air Fryer for an additional minute until the cheese melts. Yummy!

Yields: Serves Three

Pigs In A Blanket

Ingredients

1 (Eight-ounce) Can crescent rolls

1 (Twelve-ounce) Package cocktail franks

Instructions

1) Preheat the Air Fryer to 330ºF.

2) Drain the Franks and thoroughly dry them using two paper towels.

3) Slice the dough into strips of about 1 ½ inches x 1-inch (rectangular).

4) Roll the dough around the Franks leaving the ends open. Put them in the freezer to firm up for about five minutes.

5) Take them out, and put them in the AF for six to eight minutes. Adjust the temperature to 390ºF, and continue to cook for approximately three minutes.

Yields: Serves Four

Chicken

AF Chicken 'Fried.'

Ingredients

2 chicken thighs (skinless)

3 sprigs fresh parsley

Garlic powder (to dust the thighs)

Salt and black pepper if desired

½ a lemon

Chili flakes as you like

1 to 2 sprigs fresh rosemary

Instructions

1) Rinse the thighs. Drain them between two paper towels. (Discard the towels and wash your hands.)

2) Clean the rosemary sprigs and remove the stems. Chop or mince the parsley.

3) *For the Marinate*: Combine the salt and pepper, garlic powder, rosemary leaves, parsley, chili flakes, and lemon juice. Add the thighs and marinate overnight in the refrigerator.

4) *Preheat the Air Fryer*: Set the AF to 356ºF.

5) Grill for 12 minutes.

Note: Times may vary depending on the thickness/size of the thighs.

AF Buffalo Chicken Wings

Ingredients

5 chicken wings (about 14 ounces)

½ teaspoon garlic powder (optional)

2 teaspoons cayenne pepper

2 tablespoons red hot sauce

1 tablespoon (15 grams) melted butter

Fresh black pepper and salt to taste

Instructions

1) Preheat the Air Fryer at 356ºF.

2) Cut the wings into three sections (the end tip, mid joint, and drumstick). Pat each one thoroughly dry using a paper towel. Wash your wash right away to prevent cross contamination.

3) Combine a dash of pepper and salt, the garlic powder, and cayenne pepper in a plate. Lightly coat the wings with the powder.

4) Place the chicken on the wire rack and back for 15 minutes; turning once at 7 minutes.

5) Combine the hot sauce, and melted butter in a dish to garnish the baked chicken when it is time to be served.

Notes: Save and freeze the end tip for preparing the chicken stock.

You can increase the cayenne pepper if you want it hotter.

Country Style Chicken Tenders

Ingredients

¾ pounds chicken tenders

2 tablespoons olive oil

½ teaspoon salt

2 beaten eggs

½ cup all-purpose flour

½ cup seasoned breadcrumbs

1 teaspoon black pepper

Instructions

1) Preheat the Air Fryer heat to 330ºF.

2) Set up three separate dishes for the flour, eggs, and breadcrumbs.

3) Blend the salt, pepper and bread crumbs. Pour in the oil with the breadcrumbs and mix. Put the chicken tenders into the flour, and the eggs. Coat

evenly with the breadcrumbs. Shake the excess off before placing in the Air Fryer basket.

4) Cook for ten minutes at 330ºF and increase to 390ºF for five minutes or until they are a nice golden brown.

Chinese Chicken Wings

Ingredients

4 chicken wings

Salt and pepper to taste

1 tablespoon each:

- Chinese spice

- Mixed spice

- Soy sauce

Instructions

Preheat the AF to 180ºC/356ºF.

1) Add the seasonings into a large mixing container—stirring thoroughly.

2) Blend the seasonings over the chicken wings until each piece is covered.

3) Put some aluminum foil on the base of the AF (similar to how you cover a baking tray), and add the chicken sprinkling any remnants over the chicken. Cook for 15 minutes.

4) Flip the chicken and cook another 15 minutes at 200C/392F.

Yields: Two Servings

Chicken Pot Pie

Ingredients

6 chicken tenders

2 potatoes

1 ½ cups condensed cream of celery soup

¾ cup heavy cream

1 thyme sprig

1 whole dried bay leaf

5 refrigerated buttermilk biscuits (dough)

1 tablespoon milk

1 egg yolk

Instructions

1) Preheat the Air Fryer at 320ºF.

2) Peel and dice the potatoes.

3) Mix all of the ingredients in a pan except for the milk, egg yolk, and biscuits. Bring them to a boil using medium heat.

4) Empty the mixture into the baking tin and use some aluminum foil to cover the top. Place the pan into the fry basket. Set the timer for 15 minutes.

5) Meanwhile, after the pie completes the cycle make an egg wash with the milk and egg yolk. Place the biscuits on the baking pan and brush with the egg wash mixture.

6) Set the timer to 300ºF for an additional ten minutes.

7) Your pie is ready when the biscuits are golden brown.

Yields: Four Servings

Tarragon Chicken

Ingredients

1 skinless and boneless chicken breast

⅛ Teaspoon fresh ground black pepper

½ Teaspoon unsalted butter

⅛ Teaspoon kosher salt

¼ Cup dried tarragon

Instructions

1) Pre-set the cooker to 390ºF.

2) Cut a piece of heavy-duty aluminum foil—approximately 12 x 12 or you can double a regular strength one and fold in half. Put the chicken on it.

3) Place the butter and tarragon on top of the chicken and flavor with pepper and salt—loosely wrapping the chicken for minimal airflow.

4) Cook for 12 minutes in the Air Fryer basket, remove the meal from the wrapper and enjoy.

Beef

Beef Roll Ups

Ingredients

6 slices provolone cheese

2 pounds beef flank steak

3 tablespoons pesto

¾ cup fresh baby spinach

1 teaspoon each sea salt and ground black pepper

3-ounces roasted red bell peppers

Instructions

1) Preheat the Air Fryer cooker to 400ºF.

2) Open the steak up and add the butter and pesto evenly on the meat.

3) Layer in the spinach, peppers, and cheese about three-quarters the way down through the meat.

4) Roll the mixture and secure it with toothpicks or skewers.

5) Set the timer for 14 minutes; flipping the beef halfway through the cooking process.

6) Let the meat rest for a minimum of ten minutes before attempting to cut and serve the tasty delight.

Yields: Four Servings

Air Fried Ravioli

Ingredients

1 package meat or cheese ravioli

1 jar Marinara sauce

2 C. breadcrumbs (Italian-style)

1 C. buttermilk

¼ C. Parmesan cheese

Olive oil

Note: Purchase the sauce and ravioli ready-made.

Instructions

1) Preheat the Air Fryer to 200ºF.

2) Empty the buttermilk into a container and dip the ravioli.

3) Put a spoonful of oil to the breadcrumbs. Coat the ravioli with the crumbs.

4) Add the ravioli into the AF on baking paper for around five minutes.

Roasted Veggie Pasta Salad

Ingredients

4 ounces brown mushrooms

1 red onion

1 yellow squash

1 zucchini

1 each bell peppers

- Red

- Green

- Orange

Pinch of Fresh ground pepper and salt

1 teaspoon Italian seasoning

1 cup grape tomatoes

½ cup pitted Kalamata olives

1 pound cooked Rigatoni or Penne Rigate

¼ cup olive oil

2 tablespoons fresh chopped basil

3 tablespoons balsamic vinegar

Instructions

1) Cut the squash and zucchini into half-moons. Cut the peppers into large chunks and slice the red onion. Slice the tomatoes and olives in half.

2) Preheat the Air Fryer to 380ºF.

3) Put the mushrooms, peppers, red onion, squash, and zucchini in a large container.

4) Drizzle with some of the oil—tossing well. Sprinkle in the pepper, salt, and Italian seasoning.

5) Place in the Air Fryer until the veggies are soft (not mushy), usually about for 12 to 15

minutes. For even roasting; shake the basket about halfway through the cooking cycle.

6) Combine the roasted veggies, olives, cooked pasta, and tomatoes, in a large container; mix well. Add the vinegar, and toss. (Use as little oil as possible, just enough to coat the vegetables.)

7) Keep it refrigerated until ready to serve— adding the fresh basil for last.

Yields: Six to Eight Servings

Chapter 4: Air Fryer Dinner Recipes

Chicken and Turkey Recipes

Lemon Rosemary Chicken

Ingredients

1 pound chicken (350 g)

For the Marinade:

1 tablespoon soy sauce

½ tablespoon olive oil

1 teaspoon minced ginger

For the Sauce:

3 tablespoons brown sugar

1 tablespoon oyster sauce

½ wedge-cut lemon in skins

Optional: 15 g (0.5 ounces) fresh rosemary

Instructions

1) Leave the skin on the rosemary and chop.

2) Blend all of the marinade components.. Pour over the chicken. Let them cool off in the fridge for about thirty minutes.

3) Place the marinade and chicken in a baking dish, and bake for six minutes in the AF at 392ºF.

4) Blend all of the sauce ingredients (minus the lemon).

5) Pour the mixture over the chicken when it is about half baked.

6) Place the lemon wedges in the pan evenly and squeeze so the zest will heighten the flavor of the chicken. Continue baking for an additional 13 minutes turning to ensure all of the pieces are browned evenly.

Note: You can omit the rosemary.

Jamaican Chicken Meatballs

Ingredients

1 large peeled and diced onion

2 large chicken breasts

1 teaspoon chili powder

2 tablespoons honey

Pepper and salt to taste

3 tablespoons soy sauce

1 tablespoon each:

- Dry mustard
- Cumin
- Thyme
- Basil

Optional: 2 teaspoons Jerk Paste

Instructions

1) Using a blender—mince the chicken; add the onion and mince; mix well. Toss in the Jamaican seasonings and blend again. Make ten medium balls.

2) Place on the baking mat in the AF and cook at 356ºF or 180ºC.

3) Put them on a stick when done cooking and some use of the extra sauce over the meatballs.

4) Add several herbs on the top, serve, and enjoy.

Yields: Ten Servings

Note: In case you are not aware; jerk paste is a combination of brown spices, ginger, peppers, and thyme.

Roast Turkey Breast

Ingredients

1 tablespoon ground black pepper

8 pounds bone-in turkey breast

2 tablespoon each:

- Olive oil
- Sea salt

Instructions

1) Preheat the Air Fryer on 360ºF.

2) Rub the turkey with olive oil and flavor with the seasonings.

3) Put the turkey in the preheated basket for 20 minutes.

4) When done, flip it over and adjust the cooking time for another 20 minutes (also at 360ºF).

5) The breast of turkey is done when it registers 165ºF when thermometer tested.

6) Allow the meat rest a minimum of 20 minutes before serving.

Spicy Rolled Meat

Ingredients

1 (1.6 pounds/500 g) turkey breast fillet

½ tsp. chili powder

1 ½ tsp. ground cumin

1 crushed garlic clove

1 tsp. cinnamon

2 Tbsp. olive oil

1 small finely chopped onion

2 Tbsp. flat-leafed parsley (finely chopped)

Needed: Rolled meat String

Instructions

1) Preset the heat on the Air Fryer at 356ºF/180ºC.

2) Put the meat on a cutting board with the short end facing you. Cut the full length of the fillet. Stop cutting about (2 cm, 13/16inches) from

the edge and about 1/3 of the way from the top. Fold this section open and cut it again from this side and open the meat.

3) Combine the cinnamon, chili powder, 1 teaspoon of salt, pepper, and cumin in a mixing container in a small mixing container. Pour in the oil.

4) Spoon one tablespoon of the mixture into a small dish and add the parsley and onion.

5) Use the mixture to coat the meat.

6) Tie it starting at 1 ¼-inch intervals.

7) Rub the outside with the herbal mixture for about 40 minutes or until nicely browned.

Yields: Four Servings

Fish and Seafood

Salmon Patties

Ingredients

1 salmon portion (about 7 ounces)

3 large russet potatoes (about 14 ounces)

1/3 cup frozen veggies (parboiled & drained)

2 dill sprinkles

Dash of salt and pepper

1 egg

Coating: breadcrumbs

Olive oil spray

Instructions

1) Set the Air Fryer to 356ºF.

2) Peel and chop the potatoes into small bits and boil for about ten minutes.

3) Mash and place in the fridge to chill.

4) Grill the salmon for five minutes, flake it apart and set it to the side.

5) Combine all of the ingredients and shape into patties.

6) Evenly coat with the breadcrumbs, and spray them with a bit of olive spray.

7) Place in the Air Fryer for ten to twelve minutes.

Yields: Six to Eight Patties

Dill Salmon

Ingredients for the Salmon

4 (6-ounce pieces) or 1 ½ pounds salmon

1 Pinch of salt

2 Teaspoons olive oil

Ingredients for the Dill Sauce

½ cup each:

- Sour cream

- Non-fat Greek yogurt

- 2 (finely chopped) tablespoons dill

- 1 Pinch of salt

Instructions

1) Preheat the AF to 270ºF.

2) Slice the salmon into the four portions, and drizzle with half of the oil (1 teaspoon). Flavor with a pinch of salt and add to the basket for about 20 to 23 minutes.

3) *Make the Sauce*: Blend the sour cream, yogurt, salt, and dill in a mixing container. Pour the sauce over the cooked salmon as a garnish with a pinch of the chopped dill.

Yields: Serves Four

Halibut Steak With a Teriyaki Glazed Sauce

Ingredients

1 Lb. halibut steak

Ingredients for the Marinade

½ cup mirin (Japanese cooking wine)

2/3 cup low-sodium soy sauce

¼ cup sugar

¼ cup orange juice

2 tablespoons lime juice

¼ teaspoon each:

- Ground ginger
- Crushed red pepper flakes

1 smashed garlic clove

Instructions

1) Preheat the Air Fryer to 390ºF.

2) Combine all of the marinade ingredients in a saucepan, bring it to a boil and reduce to

medium heat; cool.

3) Pour half of the marinade in a resealable plastic bag with the halibut. Chill in the fridge for thirty minutes.

4) Cook the halibut for ten to twelve minutes. Brush some of the remaining glazes over the steak.

5) Serve over the top of a bed of rice. Add a little basil or mint for some extra jazz.

Yields: Serves Three

Cajun Shrimp

Ingredients

1 tablespoon olive oil

½ teaspoon Old Bay seasoning

16 to 20 (1 ¼ pounds) tiger shrimp

¼ teaspoon each:

- smoked paprika

- cayenne pepper

1 pinch of salt

Instructions

1) Preheat the Air Fryer to 390ºF.

2) Mix all of the ingredients and coat the shrimp with the oil and spices.

3) Place the shrimp in the basket and cook for five minutes.

4) Complement the meal with some rice and place the shrimp on top for a tasty luncheon treat.

Coconut Shrimp

Ingredients

12 Large raw shrimp

1 tablespoon cornstarch

½ tablespoon oil

1 Cup each:

- Raw egg whites

- Unsweetened dried coconut

- White all-purpose flour
- Panko

Instructions

1) Drain the shrimp on towels

2) Preheat the AF to 350ºF.

3) Combine the coconut and panko in a container and set it to the side; blend the cornstarch and oil in another dish.

4) Put the egg whites into another container, and a third one for the coconut mix.

5) Cover each shrimp in the cornstarch mix, the egg whites, and lastly the coconut mixture.

6) Cook for ten minutes; flipping them after five minutes for even cooking.

Yields: Three Servings

Beef

Rib Steak

Ingredients

1 Tablespoon of steak rub

2 pounds rib steaks

1 Tablespoon of olive oil

Instructions

1) Before it is time to cook; preheat the Air Fryer to 400ºF.

2) Flavor the meat on all areas with the oil and rub.

3) Put it in the basket for 14 minutes, flipping after seven minutes.

4) Let it rest for at least ten minutes before you slice and serve.

Yields: Two Servings

Stromboli

Ingredients

1 (12-ounce) refrigerated pizza crust

¾ cup Mozzarella shredded cheese

3 cups shredded cheddar cheese

1 tablespoon milk

1 egg yolk

1/3 pound sliced cooked ham

3 ounces roasted red bell peppers

Instructions

1) Preheat the Air Fryer at 360ºF.

2) Roll the dough until it is around ¼-inch thick.

3) Layer in the peppers, ham, and cheese on one side of the dough and fold to seal.

4) Combine the milk and eggs to brush the dough.

5) Put the Stromboli in the basket and set the timer for 15 minutes. Check it every five minutes or so— flip the Stromboli to the other side for thorough cooking.

Yields: Four Servings

Roasted Rack of Lamb with a Macadamia Crust

Ingredients

1 clove of garlic

1 Tbsp. olive oil

Pepper and salt

1 ¾ pounds - rack of lamb

Ingredients for the Crust

3 ounces Macadamia nuts (unsalted)

1 tablespoon each

- Fresh rosemary

- Breadcrumbs

1 egg

Instructions

1) Preheat the Air Fryer to 220ºF.

2) Chop the garlic clove into tiny bits. Make the garlic oil by combining the garlic and oil. Brush the lamb and flavor with salt and pepper.

3) Chop the nuts to a fine consistency in a bowl and blend in the rosemary and breadcrumbs. Beat/whip the egg in another dish.

4) Dredge the meat in the egg mixture and coat with the macadamia crust topping.

5) Place the rack of lamb in the Air Fryer basket —setting the timer for 30 minutes.

6) After the time is lapsed; raise the heat to 390ºF—setting the time for an additional five minutes.

7) Take the meat from the fryer and let it rest for about ten minutes covered with some aluminum foil.

Substitutes: You can use cashews, hazelnuts, pistachios, or almonds if you would like a change of pace.

Crispy Tofu

Ingredients

2 tsp. toasted sesame oil

2 Tbsp. soy sauce

1 tsp. seasoned rice vinegar

1 block firm pressed tofu

1 tablespoon cornstarch or potato starch

Instructions

1) Cut the tofu into 1-inch cubes. Preheat the Air Fryer to 370ºF.

2) In a shallow dish, mix the vinegar, soy sauce,

oil, and tofu. Let the combination marinate for 15 to 30 minutes. Toss the marinated product with the cornstarch and add it to the AF basket.

3) Cook for 20 minutes, shaking the basket halfway through the cooking cycle.

Yields: Four Servings

Sides

Bread Rolls with Potato Stuffing

Ingredients

8 slices bread (white part only)

5 large potatoes

1 small bunch finely chopped coriander

2 seeded and finely chopped green chilies

½ teaspoon turmeric

2 curry leaf sprigs

½ teaspoon mustard seeds

2 finely chopped small onions

2 tablespoons oil (frying and brushing)

Salt if desired

Instructions

1) Preheat the Air Fryer to 392ºF.

2) Cut away the edges of the bread.

3) Peel the potatoes, and boil. Use one teaspoon of salt, and mash the potatoes.

4) In the meantime, on the stovetop using a skillet to combine the mustard seeds and one teaspoon of the oil. Add the onions when the seeds sputter, continue frying until they become translucent. Toss in the curry and turmeric.

5) Fry the mixture a few seconds, then add the salt, mashed potatoes; mix well, and let it cool.

6) Shape eight portions of the mixture into an oval shape. Set to the side.

7) Wet the bread with water, and press it into your palm to remove the excess water.

8) Place the oval potato into the bread and roll the bread completely around the potato mixture. Be sure they are completely sealed.

9) Brush the basket and the potato rolls with oil, and set to the side.

10) Set the Air Fryer timer for 12 to 13 minutes. Let them cook until crispy and browned.

Yields: Four Servings

Avocado Fries

Ingredients

1 large avocado

Pinch of black pepper and salt

¼ teaspoon paprika or cayenne pepper

¼ cup all-purpose flour

½ cup Panko breadcrumbs

1 beaten egg

¼ of a lemon

Instructions

1) Preheat the Air Fryer to 392ºF.

2) Cut the avocado into eight slices.

3) Using three separate containers; add the salt, cayenne, pepper, and flour in one. Place the beaten egg in the second one and breadcrumbs in the third one.

4) Coat the avocado with the flour, egg, and breadcrumbs.

5) Put the avocado into the fryer basket and set the timer for six minutes.

6) They will be golden in color when ready to serve.

Enjoy with some Greek yogurt and honey or with a squeeze of fresh lemon juice.

Broccoli

Ingredients

2 Lbs. broccoli crowns .

2 Tablespoons olive oil

1 teaspoon kosher salt

½ teaspoon black pepper

2 teaspoons grated lemon zest

1/3 cup Kalamata olives

¼ cup shaved Parmesan cheese

Instructions

1) Remove the stems from the broccoli and cut

them into 1 to 1-1/2- inch florets. Pit and cut

the olives in half.

2) Over high heat, fill a medium pan with six cups

of water—bring it to boiling. Toss in the florets

and cook for three to four minutes. Remove

and drain. Add the pepper, salt, and oil

3) Set the AF to 400ºF.

4) Place the broccoli into the basket, close the

drawer, and click the timer for 15 minutes.

Toss/flip at seven minutes for even browning.

When done, place the broccoli in the bowl.

5) Garnish with lemon zest, olives, and cheese.

Enjoy immediately.

Yields: Two to Four Servings

Fact: The Kalamata olive is a native of southern Greece

which is often times preserved in olive oil or wine

vinegar. It is an additional 'kick' for this treat!

Buffalo Cauliflower

Ingredients

1 cup breadcrumbs

4 cups cauliflower florets

¼cup buffalo sauce

¼ cup melted butter

For the Dip: Your favorite dressing

Instructions

1) Place the butter in a microwaveable dish; remove and whisk in the buffalo sauce.

2) Dip each of the florets in the buttery mixture; the stem does not need to have sauce. Use the stem as a handle, hold it over a cup and let the excess drip away.

3) Run the floret through the breadcrumbs to your liking. Drop them into the fryer. Cook for 14 to 17 minutes at 350ºF. (The unit will not need to preheat since it is calculated at the time.)

4) You can shake the basket several times to be sure it is evenly browning. Enjoy with your

favorite dip, but be sure to eat it right away because the crunchiness goes away quickly.

Note: Reheat in the oven. Don't reheat it in the microwave; it will be mushy.

Yields: Four Servings

Cheesy Potatoes

Ingredients

7 medium potatoes

½ cup grated Gruyere (semi-mature) cheese

½ cup cream

½cup milk

1 teaspoon black pepper

½ teaspoon nutmeg

Instructions

1) Peel and slice the potatoes wafer-thin. Russet potatoes work great with this recipe.

2) Preset the Air Fryer to 400ºF.

3) Blend the milk and cream; add the nutmeg pepper, and salt for seasoning.

4) Generously coat the potatoes with the mixture.

5) Put the slices in an 8 x 8 dish, pouring the rest of the mixture over the potatoes.

6) Place the dish into Air Fryer and set the timer for 25 minutes.

7) Remove the dish and sprinkle the cheese over the hot potatoes.

8) Continue cooking until the cheese is melted and browned, usually an additional ten minutes.

Yields: Serves Six

French Fried Potatoes

Ingredients

6 medium peeled potatoes

2 Tbsp. olive oil

Instructions

1) Preheat the Air Fryer to 360ºF.

2) Peel and cut the potatoes into 3-inch strips x ¼-inch.

3) Soak the cut potatoes for a minimum of thirty minutes in water, and drain thoroughly. Pat

them dry with a towel.

4) Coat the potatoes with the oil .in a large mixing container. .

5) Drop the potatoes into the cooking basket. for about thirty minutes or until they are the desired doneness.

6) Shake the basket two or three times during the cooking phase.

Note: The time may vary depending on the thickness of the potatoes.

Potatoes Au Gratin

Ingredients

7 Medium peeled russet potatoes

½ cup each:

- Cream

- Milk

½ teaspoon nutmeg

1 teaspoon black pepper

½ cup semi-mature (Gruyere) grated cheese

Instructions

1) Preheat the Air Fryer to 390ºF.

2) Wash and slice the potatoes wafer-thin.

3) Blend together the cream and milk—flavoring with some pepper, salt, and nutmeg.

4) Use the milk mixture to coat the potatoes.

5) Place the slices into an eight-inch baking pan/ dish and pour the remainder of the milk/cream mixture on top of the potatoes.

6) Place the heat-resistant dish onto the cooking basket—setting the timer for 25 minutes.

7) Take the basket out and sprinkle with the cheese.

8) Bake ten more minutes or until browned.

Note: You can use two eggs instead of milk.

Yields: Six Servings

Homemade AF Croutons

Try these with a healthy salad:

Ingredients

Stale Bread

Butter

Optional: Olive oil

Instructions

1) Preheat the Air Fryer for about two to three minutes at 248ºF. (You can always adjust the time but don't hotter than 320ºF.)

2) Cube some of the old bread to the sizes you want to use for your meal. Pour in the olive oil and melted butter.

3) Put the cubed bread in the basket and cook for two to three minutes.

4) Toss and cook for an additional two to three minutes.

5) Completely cool and keep in an airtight container for no more than two days.

Portobello Mushrooms

Ingredients

1.4 Oz. cubed ham (about two slices)

4 Tbsp. extra virgin olive oil

7.05 Oz. Portobello mushrooms

2 shiitake or button mushrooms

1.8 Oz. Mozzarella cheese (shredded)

1 Tbsp. chopped garlic

Optional: Ground black pepper and salt

Instructions

1) Preheat the AF cooker at 356ºF.

2) Clean, cap, and remove the stalks from the mushrooms; use a couple of paper towels to pat them dry.

3) Use 1/2 of the oil to brush the Portobello mushrooms tops and place them cap side down on a baking tray lined with aluminum foil or parchment paper.

4) Divide the mushrooms and top with cheese, garlic, the other half of mushrooms—diced, and the cubed ham.

5) Flavor with the pepper and salt. Drizzle a bit of the oil over the mushrooms.

6) Cook for about 10 minutes. Garnish with some dried or fresh parsley.

The Blooming Onion

Ingredients

4 small/medium onions

4 dollops of butter

1 Tbsp. olive oil

Instructions

1) Peel the skin from the onion and cut away the top and bottom to reveal flat ends.

2) Soak the onions in salt water for four hours to take away the harshness.

3) You'll need to cut the onion as far down as you can without severing the onion. Cut four times to make eight segments.

4) Preheat the fryer to 350ºF.

5) Put the onions in the fryer and drizzle with the oil —placing a dollop of butter on each one.

6) Cook in the AF until the outside is dark, usually about thirty minutes.

Note: 4 dollops is 4 heaping tablespoons

Yields: Four Servings

Onion Rings

Ingredients

For a side dish or quick snack; purchase four ounces of frozen, battered onion rings.

Instructions

1) Preheat the Air Fryer cooker to 360ºF.

2) Place the frozen onion rings in the basket for ten minutes.

3) Take them from the cooker and give them a toss.

4) Reset the timer for an additional ten minutes or more if needed.

Fat-Free Fries

Ingredients

1 to 2 sweet potatoes

1 to 2 red potatoes

Sprinkle of pepper and salt

Cooking spray

Optional: Parsley

Instructions

1) Preset the Air Fryer for 356ºF.

2) Peel and cut the potatoes; place in a container of water until ready for frying.

3) Use two layers of paper towels to dry the wedges and spray them with the oil.

4) Place a single layer of fries in the basket and set the timer for ten minutes.

5) After the time is up, give the fries a shake, return to the AF for an additional eight to ten minutes.

6) Take them from the fryer and season as you wish. Garnish with a bit of parsley.

Potato Croquets

Ingredients

7 small cubed red potatoes

1 egg yolk

2 Tablespoons all-purpose flour

½ cup grated Parmesan cheese

1 Pinch Each:

- Cayenne

- Black pepper

- Salt

For the Breading:

1 cup all-purpose flour

2 Tablespoons vegetable oil

2 beaten eggs

½ cup panko

1 Pinch of nutmeg

Instructions

1) Preset the temperature on the Air Fryer to 390ºF.

2) In salted water, boil the potatoes for 15 minutes, drain, and mash. Cool completely.

3) Add the flour, cheese, and egg yolk—flavoring with nutmeg, pepper, and salt,

4) Shape the filling into golf ball size.

5) Make a crumbly mixture of the breadcrumbs and oil. Put each ball into the flour mixture, the eggs, and then the panko. Roll them into cylinder shapes.

6) Put them in the cooking basket until browned —about seven to eight minutes.

Yields: It will probably take 2 batches depending on how large you made the balls.

Potato Skin Wedges

Ingredients

6 medium russet potatoes

1 ½ tsp. paprika

½ tsp. salt

2 Tbsp. canola oil

½ tsp. black pepper

Instructions

1) Thoroughly wash the potatoes under the tap. Boil the potatoes in salted water about forty minutes.

2) Cool in the refrigerator for about thirty minutes. Quarter them when cooled.

3) Combine the paprika, pepper, salt, and oil in a mixing dish. Toss the potatoes in the mixture.

4) Place in the cooking basket with the skin side down. Cook them until golden brown; about 14 to 16 minutes.

Grilled Tomatoes AF Style

Ingredients

2 tomatoes

Cooking spray

Pepper

Herbs

Instructions

1) Preheat the fryer to 320ºF.

2) Wash and cut the tomatoes into halves. Spray each of them lightly with some cooking spray and place them cut side facing upwards. Sprinkle with your favorite spices—fresh or dried—including the pepper, sage, rosemary, basil, oregano, and any others of your choice.

3) Put them into the basket for 20 minutes or until they are to the doneness you want to achieve. If they are ready to enjoy—if not—cook for a few more minutes.

This would be tasty breakfast or as a side dish.

Yields: Two Servings

Chapter 5: Air Fryer Desserts

Blackberry Apricot Crumble

Ingredients

5 ½ ounces fresh blackberries

2 tablespoons lemon juice

18 ounces fresh apricots

½ cup sugar

Pinch of salt

1 cup flour

5 tablespoons cold butter

Instructions

1) Preheat the Air Fryer to 390ºF.

2) Prepare an eight-inch oven dish with a small amount of cooking oil.

3) Remove the stones, cut the apricots into cubes, and place them in a container.

4) Mix the lemon juice, blackberries, and 2 tablespoons of sugar with the apricots and mix. Place the fruit in the oven dish.

5) Combine a pinch of salt, the remainder of the sugar, and the flour in a mixing container. Add 1 tablespoon cold water and the butter; using your fingertips to make a crumbly mixture.

6) Sprinkle the crumbles over the fruit and press down.

7) Place the dish into the basket and slide it into the Air Fryer for 20 minutes. It is ready when it is cooked thoroughly, and the top is browned.

Cheesecake: Lemon Ricotta

Ingredients

1 lemon

$^2/^3$ cups (150g) sugar

2 cups (500g) ricotta

2 teaspoons vanilla essence

Instructions

1) Zest and juice the lemon.

2) Preset the Air Fryer to 320ºF.

3) Mix the sugar, ricotta, 1 tablespoon lemon juice as well as the zest, and the vanilla essence—stirring until fully mixed. Blend in the cornstarch and pour into the oven dish.

4) Place the dish in the Air Fryer basket and set the timer for 25 minutes.

5) The middle should be set when the cake is completely done.

6) Leave the cheesecake on a wire rack to fully cool.

Cherry Pie

Ingredients

2 refrigerated pre-made pie crusts

1 Can cherry pie filling (21-ounces)

1 tablespoon milk

1 egg yolk

Instructions

1) Preheat the fryer to 310ºF.

2) Stab holes into the crust after placing into a pie plate. Allow the excess to hang over the edges. Place in the AF for five minutes

3) Take the basket out and set the crust on the counter. Fill it with the cherries. Remove the excess crust.

4) Cut the remainder crust into ¾-inch strips placing them as a lattice across the pie.

5) Make an egg wash with the milk and egg; brush the pie.

6) Bake for fifteen minutes.

7) Serve with the ice cream of your choice.

Yields: Eight Servings

Donut Bread Pudding

Ingredients

6 glazed donuts

4 raw egg yolks

1 ½ cups whipping cream

¼ cup sugar

¾ cup frozen sweet cherries

1 teaspoon cinnamon

½ cup semi-sweet chocolate baking chips

½ cup raisins

Instructions

1) Preheat the fryer at 310ºF.

2) Combine the wet ingredients in a container and combine the rest of the ingredients and mix.

3) Pour into a baking pan and cover it with foil. Place it into the basket and set the timer for 60 minutes.

4) Chill the bread pudding well before serving.

Yields: Four Servings

Fluffy Peanut Butter Marshmallow Turnovers

Ingredients

4 defrosted sheets filo pastry

4 Tbsp. chunky peanut butter

2-ounces melted butter

4 tsp. marshmallow fluff

A Pinch of sea salt

Instructions

1) Preset the temperature of the Air Fryer to 360ºF.

2) Use the melted butter to brush one sheet of the filo. Put the second sheet on top and brush it also with butter.

3) Continue the process until you have completed all four sheets.

4) Cut the layers into four (4) 12-inch x 3-inch strips.

5) Place one teaspoon of the marshmallow fluff on the underside and 1 tablespoon of the peanut butter.

6) Fold the tip over the filo strip to form a triangle, making sure the filling is completely wrapped.

7) Seal the ends with a small amount of butter. Place the completed turnovers into the AF for three to five minutes.

8) When done, they will be fluffy and golden brown.

9) Add a touch of sea salt for the sweet/salty combo.

Notes: The Filo/Phyllo pastry is a little different than regular pastry. It is tissue thin and has very little fat content. It is considered okay by some bakers and is interchange the filo with regular puff pastry for turnovers.

Yields: Four Servings

Marshmallow and Yam Hand Pies

Ingredients

1 crescent dough sheet

1 (16-ounce can) candied yams

1/2 teaspoon cinnamon

1/4 teaspoon allspice

2 tablespoons marshmallow crème

1/4 teaspoon salt

1 egg, beaten

For the Maple Glaze:

1/2 cup maple syrup

½ cup confectioners' sugar

Instructions

1) Pre-set the heat on the AF to 400ºF.

2) Drain the syrup from the yams. Combine the cinnamon, salt, allspice, and yams using a fork to the blend the spices and mash the yams.

3) Put the dough sheet onto a board and cut into four equal sections.

4) Spoon the filling onto the squares and add a tablespoon of the crème.

5) Use a brush to spread the egg over the edges of the dough and place the remainder of the two pieces of dough on top of the pies.

6) Use a fork to crimp the edges and cut three slits in the top for venting.

7) Place in the Air Fryer for six minutes.

8) Make the glaze from the sugar and syrup in a small dish—slowly adding the syrup—until the sugar dissolves.

9) To serve, drizzle the glaze over the warm pies and enjoy.

Yields: Four Servings.

Orange and Pineapple Fondant

Ingredients

4.2 ounces (115) g Butter

4.2 ounces (115 g) Dark chocolate

2 medium eggs

4 tablespoons castor sugar (see note below)

2 tablespoons self-rising flour

1 medium orange (rind and juice)

Instructions

1) Grease four ramekins with a small amount of oil or cooking spray.

2) Pre-set the heat in the Air Fryer to 356ºF/380ºC.

3) Cut and tear apart the orange and grate the orange peel.

4) Melt the butter and chocolate in a double boiler or in a glass measuring cup over a pot of hot water. Stir until it is creamy smooth.

5) Beat and whisk in the sugar and eggs—until frothy and pale. Blend in the sugar and egg mixture along with the orange bits. Add the flour and mix until well-blended.

6) Fill the ramekins about ¾ of the way full with the mixture. Cook in the Air Fryer for 12

minutes.

7) Take it from the fryer and let them rest for two minutes. (They will continue to cook.) Turn them out of the containers (upside down) into a serving platter. You can loosen the edges by tapping the ramekin gently with a butter knife.

8) The fondant will release from the center to provide you with a luscious center of pudding.

9) Garnish with some caramel sauce or vanilla ice cream.

Yields: Four Servings

How to Make Castor Sugar

Castor or caster sugar is simply granulated sugar that has been placed into a blender or food processor to make it a 'super-fine' sugar used for some recipes since it melts easier.

Instructions

1) Put the granulated sugar into the blender/food

processor.

2) Pulse until it is a 'super-fine' texture—not powdery.

Pineapple Sticks with Yogurt Dip

Ingredients

¼ C. desiccated (moisture-free) coconut

1 C. vanilla yogurt

1 small sprig fresh mint

Instructions

1) Preheat the Air Fryer to 392ºF.

2) Meanwhile, use similar shapes and sizes to cut the pineapple into sticks.

3) Dip the sticks into the coconut. Place the pineapple sticks in the basket and cook for ten minutes

4) *For the Dip*: Dice the mint into the yogurt.

Yields: Four Servings

Strawberry Cupcakes and Strawberry Icing

Ingredients

½ cup castor sugar

½ cup butter

2 medium eggs

½ cup self-rising flour

½ cup butter

½ teaspoon vanilla essence

½ cup icing sugar

1 tablespoon whipped cream

½ teaspoon pink food coloring

¼ cup fresh (blended) strawberries

Instructions

1) Set the Air Fryer temperature to 338ºF/170ºC.

2) Cream the sugar and butter in a large mixing container until it is creamy smooth.

3) Add the eggs one at a time along with the vanilla essence.

4) Blend in a small amount of flour at a time until all is completely mixed.

5) Pour them into ramekins about 80% of the way full. Place them in the Air Fryer for eight minutes.

6) *Make the Frosting:* Cream the butter and slowly mix in the icing sugar until creamy. Pour in the food coloring, (blended) strawberries, and whipped cream—mix well.

7) Take them out and use a piping bag to make the swirly frosting for a tasty 'pretty' cupcake every time.

Yields: Ten Servings

Chapter 6: Air Fryer Appetizers and Snacks

Cheesy Garlic Bread

Ingredients

5 round bread slices

5 teaspoons sun-dried tomato pesto

3 chopped garlic cloves

4 Tbsp. melted butter

1 cup grated Mozzarella cheese

Garnish Options:

- Chili flakes

- Chopped basil leaves

- oregano

Instructions

1) Preheat the Air Fryer to 356ºF.

2) Cut the loaf of bread into 5 thick slices.

3) Add the butter, pesto, and cheese on the bread.

4) Put the slices in the preheated cooker for six to eight minutes.

5) Garnish with your choice of toppings.

Note: Round or Baguette bread was used for this recipe. It is recommended to add the finely chopped garlic cloves to the melted butter ahead of time for the best results.

Clams Oregano

Ingredients

2 dozen shucked clams

1 cup unseasoned breadcrumbs

4 tablespoons melted butter

3 clove minced garlic

1 teaspoon dried oregano

¼ cup chopped parsley

¼ cup grated Parmesan cheese

For the Pan:

- 1 cup sea salt

Instructions

1) Preheat the AF to 400ºF.

2) Mix the oregano, parsley, parmesan cheese, breadcrumbs, and melted butter in a medium container.

3) Using a heaping tablespoon of the crumb mixture; add it to the exposed clams.

4) Fill the insert with the salt, place the clams inside and cook for three minutes.

5) Dress them up with a garnish of lemon wedges and fresh parsley.

Yields: Four Servings

Corn Tortilla Chips

Ingredients

8 corn Tortillas

1 Tbsp. olive oil

Salt if desired

Instructions

1) Preset the AF to 392ºF.

2) Use a sharp knife to cut the tortillas.

3) Brush each tortilla with oil.

4) Air fry two batches for three minutes each. Sprinkle with a pinch of salt.

Crab Sticks

Ingredients

1 package 'DoDo' crab sticks

Cooking spray

Instructions

1) Take each of the sticks out of the package; find an edge, and unroll until flat.

2) Tear the sheets into 1/3 widths.

3) Place them on a plate and coat them with cooking spray.

4) Cook them in the AF for 10 minutes.

5) *Note*: If you shred the crab meat; you can cut the time in half, but they will also easily fall through the holes in the basket.

Garlic Knots

Ingredients

Marinara sauce

1 teaspoon sea salt

1 Lb. frozen pizza crust dough

1 tablespoon each:

- Garlic powder

- Grated Parmesan cheese

- Fresh chopped parsley

Instructions

1) Preheat the Air Fryer to 360ºF.

2) Roll out the dough until is about 1 ½ to 2-inches thick. Slice it approximately ¾-inches apart—lengthwise.

3) Roll the dough and make it into knots.

4) Add the cheese, oil, and spices in a bowl, and roll each knot in the mixture before placing it into the fry basket.

5) Set the timer for 12 minutes; flipping halfway through the cooking process (six minutes).

Serve with a dish of marinara sauce.

Yields: Four Servings

Kale Chips

Ingredients

1 Tbsp. olive oil

1 head of kale

1 tsp. Soya sauce

Instructions

1) De-stem the kale and tear it into 1 1/2 –inch pieces.

2) Rinse in cold water and thoroughly dry using some paper towels.

3) Toss the kale with the soya sauce and oil.

4) Set the Air Fryer for 200ºF for two to three minutes; toss when half cooked.

Meatballs for the Party

Ingredients

2 ½ Tablespoons Worcestershire sauce

1 pound ground beef

1 Tablespoon Tabasco

¾ cup tomato ketchup

1 Tablespoon lemon juice

¼ cup vinegar

½ teaspoon dry mustard

½ cup brown sugar

3 crushed gingersnaps

Instructions

1) Combine all of the seasonings in a large mixing container—blending well.

2) Mix the beef and continue churning the ingredients.

3) Make the balls and put them in the fryer. Cook on 375ºF for 15 minutes.

4) Place them on the toothpicks before serving.

Note: They are ready when the center is done, and they are crispy.

Yields: 24 Servings

Feta Triangles

Ingredients

4 ounces feta cheese

1 egg yolk

2 tablespoons finely chopped flat-leafed parsley

2 sheets frozen (defrosted) filo pastry

1 finely chopped scallion

2 tablespoons olive oil

Ground black pepper

Instructions

1) Pre-set the heat in the Air Fryer to 390ºF.

2) Whisk the egg and blend in the scallion, feta, and parsley.

3) Cut the dough into three strips.

4) Place a heaping teaspoon of the feta mix underneath the pastry strip.

5) Fold the tip to form a triangle as you work your way around the strip.

6) Use a small amount of oil and brush each of the triangles before placing them in the cooker basket cooking them for three minutes.

7) Lower the heat to 360ºF, and continue cooking for an additional two minutes.

Yields: Five Servings

Mozzarella Sticks

Ingredients

2 eggs

1 pound or block Mozzarella cheese

1 cup plain breadcrumbs

¼ cup white flour

3 tablespoons nonfat milk

Instructions

1) Preheat the fryer to 400ºF.

2) Slice the cheese into ½-inch x 3-inch sticks.

3) Whisk the milk and egg together in one bowl, with the oil and bread crumbs in individual dishes as well.

4) Dredge the sliced cheese through the oil, egg, and breadcrumbs.

5) Place the sticks on bread tin and put them in the freezer compartment for about an hour or two.

6) Place them in small increments (don't overcrowd) into the AF basket.

7) Cook for 12 minutes.

Yields: Four Servings

Mini Quiche Wedges

Ingredients

1 (3 ½ ounces or 100 g) Frozen or ready-made pizza crust

1 egg

(1.4 ounces or 40 g) Grated cheese

½ tablespoon oil

3 tablespoons whipping cream

Fresh ground pepper

2 small pie molds

Instructions

1) Pre-set the heat on the Air Fryer to 392ºF/200ºC.

2) Use a bit of cooking spray to grease the molds. Line them with the dough pressing down around the edges.

3) Whisk the cheese, cream, and egg flavoring with some pepper and salt to taste. Empty the mixture into the molds.

4) Put the mold into the basket and set the timer for 12 minutes. Bake the second one the same way.

5) Take them from the molds and slice each of the quiches into six wedges.

6) You can serve at room temperature or warm.

Try these Variations:

Ingredients for Mushroom Slices

4.4 ounces or 125 g sliced mushrooms

1 teaspoon paprika

1 crushed clove of garlic

OR

Ingredients Ham and Broccoli

1.8 ounces or 50 g small broccoli florets and ham

Instructions for Ham and Broccoli

Boil the florets until tender.

Divide between each of the quiches.

Yields: Nine Servings

Spicy Pumpkin Patch Cannoli Treats for Halloween

Ingredients

4 tablespoons melted butter

8 large flour tortillas

1 cup sugar

½ cup orange sanding sugar

2 pounds whole milk ricotta

1 tablespoon ground cinnamon

2/3 cup confectioners' sugar

1 ½ cup pumpkin pie mix

½ cup mini chocolate chips

Instructions

1) Preheat the Air Fryer for three minutes at 400ºF.

2) Use a pumpkin cookie cutter to make the tortillas.

3) Brush one side of the cutouts with the butter and sprinkle them with the orange sanding sugar.

4) Mix the cinnamon a regular sugar in a small dish; sprinkle over the cookies.

5) Bake the treats in batches until crispy (about three minutes).

6) Use wire racks for cooling.

7) Make the dip by using a large bowl and combining the cinnamon sugar, pumpkin pie, mix, and ricotta in a large mixing dish. Stir well.

8) Be creative and place the dip in a shallow serving platter.

9) Place the crisps into the dip to make a pumpkin patch and decorate with the chips.

Yields: Four Servings

Sweet Potato Chips

Ingredients

2 Large Sweet Potatoes

1 Tbsp. olive oil

Instructions

1) Pre-set the heat in the Air Fryer to 350ºF.
2) Peel and slice the potatoes into chips. It is best to slice them into the same sizes so then will cook evenly.
3) Place the potatoes into a resealable baggie and add the oil. Shake the potatoes to coat them completely.
4) Pour the sweet potatoes into the Air Fryer and cook for approximately fifteen minutes, depending on the thickness.

PART 4

CHAPTER 1: KETO BASICS

BENEFITS OF INCREASED METABOLISM

One of the best ways to learn the meaning of a
scientific term is to break it down to its roots. When
we break down ketogenic, we see it is comprised of
two words: keto and genic. Ketones are fat-based
molecules that the body breaks down when it is
using fat as its energy source. When used as a
suffix, "genic" means "causing, forming, or
producing." So, we put these terms together, and we
have "ketogenic," or simply put, "causing fat burn."
Ergo, the theory behind ketogenic dieting is: when a
person reduces the amount of sugar and
carbohydrates they consume, the body will begin to
breakdown fat it already has in stores all over the
body. When your body is cashing in on these stores,
it is in a ketogenic state, or "ketosis." When your
body consumes food, it naturally seeks
carbohydrates for the purpose of breaking them

down and using them as fuel. Adversely, a ketogenic cleanse trains your body to use fats for energy instead. This is achieved by lowering the amount of ingested carbohydrates and increasing the amount of ingested fats, which in turn boosts your metabolism.

Only recently has a low carb- high-fat diet plan emerged into the public eye. It is a sharp contrast to the traditional dieting style that emphasizes calorie counting. For many years it was overlooked that crash diets neglect the most important aspect of dieting: food is fuel. A diet is not meant to be treated as a once a year go to method in order to shed holiday weight in January. Rather, a diet is a lifestyle; it is a consistent pattern of how individual fuels their body. A ten day ketogenic cleanse is the perfect way to begin forming healthy eating habits that over time become second nature. If you are tired of losing weight just to gain it all back, never fear. We firmly believe that you can accomplish anything you put your mind to, including living a healthy life! You, like hundreds of others, can successfully accomplish a ketogenic cleanse and change the way you see health, fitness, and life along the way. So let's hit the books and get that metabolism working!

BENEFITS OF CLEANSING

In addition to increased metabolism and fat loss, ketogenic cleansing allows your body naturally rid itself of harmful toxins and wasteful substances. In today's modern world, food is overrun and polluted by genetically modified hormones, artificial flavors and coloring, and copious amounts of unnecessary sugars. Ketogenic cleansing eliminates bread, grains, and many other foods that are most affected by today's modern industrialization. Due to the high amount of naturally occurring foods used in a ketogenic cleanse, the body is able to obtain many vitamins and minerals that are not prevalent in a high carb diet. When the body is consuming sufficient amounts of necessary vitamins and minerals, it is able to heal itself and maintain a healthy immune system. Cleansing your body is one of the best ways to achieve, and maintain pristine health.

CHAPTER 2: MEAL PLAN MADNESS

One of the best ways to stay motivated, when dieting, is to find a meal plan that is easy to follow and easy on the budget. Ketogenic meals are designed to be filling while keeping within the perimeters of low-carb, high-fat guidelines. Ideally, you want to aim for 70% fats, 25% protein, and 5% carbohydrates in your diet. As long as the materials you use to build your meals are low in carbs and high in fats, feel free to experiment and find what is right for you. Each and every one of us is different, and that's okay. After all, this meal plan is for YOU!

Below is a ten-day meal plan, designed with a busy schedule in mind, which will not break the bank! All of these meals can be prepared in 30 minutes or less, and many of them are much quicker than that! There is also a list of ingredients for each meal located in the recipe chapter so you can go to the grocery store knowing exactly what you need!

	Breakfast	Lunch	Dinner
Day 1	**California Chicken Omelet** • Fat: 32 grams • 10 minutes to prepare • Protein: 25 grams • 10 minutes of cooking • Net carbs: 4 grams	**Cobb Salad** • Fat: 48 grams • 10 minutes to prepare • Protein: 43 grams • 0 minutes of cooking • Net carbs: 3 grams	**Chicken Peanut Pad Thai** • Fat: 12 grams • 15 minutes to prepare • Protein: 30 grams • 15 minutes of cooking • Net carbs: 2 grams
Day 2	**Easy Blender Pancakes** • Fat: 29 grams • 5	**Sardine Stuffed Avocados** • Fat: 29 grams • 10 minutes to prepare	**Chipotle Fish Tacos** • Fat: 20 grams • 5 minutes to prepare • Protein:

	minutes to prepare • Protein: 41 grams • 10 minutes of cooking • Net carbs: 4 grams	• Protein: 27 grams • 0 minutes of cooking • Net Carbs: 5 grams	24 grams • 15 minutes of cooking • Net carbs: 5 grams
Day 3	**Steak and Eggs** • Fat: 36 grams • 10 minutes to prepare • Protein: 47 grams • 5 minutes of cooking • Net carbs: 3 grams	**Low-Carb Smoothie Bowl** • Fat 35 grams • 5 minutes to prepare • Protein: 20 grams • 0 minutes of cooking • Net carbs: 5 grams	**Avocado Lime Salmon** • Fat: 27 grams • 20 minutes to prepare • Protein: 37 grams • 10 minutes of cooking • Net carbs: 5 grams
KEEP IT UP!!!	During the course of your plan, especially around days 3 and 4, you may begin to feel like you don't have it in you. You may have thoughts telling you that you cannot last for ten days on this type pf cleanse. Do not allow feelings of discouragement bother you because guess what? We all feel that way		

	sometimes! A ketogenic diet causes your body to process energy like it never has before. Keep pressing on! Your body will thank you and so will you!		
Day 4	**Low-Carb Smoothie Bowl** • Fat: 35 grams • 5 minutes to prepare • Protein: 35 grams • 0 minutes of cooking • Net carbs: 4 grams	**Pesto Chicken Salad** • Fat: 27 grams • 5 minutes to prepare • Protein: 27 grams • 10 minutes of cooking • Net carbs: 3 grams	**Sriracha Lime Flank Steak** • Fat: 32 grams • 5 minutes to prepare • Protein: 48 grams • 10 minutes of cooking • Net Carbs: 5 grams
Day 5	**Feta and Pesto Omelet** • Fat: 46 grams • 5 minutes of preparation • Protein: 30 grams • 5 minutes of cooking • Net carbs: 2.5 grams	**Roasted Brussel Sprouts** • Fat: 21 grams • 5 minutes to prepare • Protein: 21 grams • 30 minut	**Low carb Sesame Chicken** • Fat: 36 grams • 15 minutes to prepare • Protein: 41 grams • 15 minut

		es of cooking • Net carbs: 4 grams	es of cooking • Net carbs: 4 grams
Day 6	**Raspberry Cream Crepes** • Fat: 40 grams • 5 minutes of preparation • Net carbs: 8 grams • 15 minutes of cooking • Protein 15 grams	**Shakshuka** • Fat: 34 grams • Protein 35 grams • Net carbs: 4 grams • 10 minutes of preparation • 10 minutes of cooking	**Sausage in a Pan** • Fat: 38 grams • 10 minutes of preparation • Protein: 30 grams • 25 minutes of cooking • Net Carbs: 4 grams
Day 7	**Green Monster Smoothie** • Fat: 25 grams • 5 minutes of preparation • Protein: 30 grams • 0 minutes of cooking • Net Carbs: 3 grams	**Tuna Tartare** • Fat: 24 grams • 15 minutes of preparation • Protein: 56 grams • 0 minutes of	**Pesto Chicken Salad** • Fat: 27 grams • 5 minutes of preparation • Protein: 27 grams • 10 minutes of

| | | cooking
• Net Carbs: 4 grams | cooking
• Net carbs: 3 grams |
|---|---|---|---|
| **ALMO ST THERE !!** | By now, you can be certain you are seeing physical results such as reduced body fat and more energy! You are doing a fantastic job, and you only have three days left! Keep up the good work; you owe it to yourself. | | |
| Day 8 | **Shakshuka**
• Fat: 34 grams
• 10 minutes of preparation
• Protein 35 grams
• 10 minutes of cooking
• Net carbs: 4 grams | **Grilled Halloumi Salad**
• Fat: 47 grams
• 15 minutes of preparation
• Protein: 21 grams
• 0 minutes of cooking
• Net carbs: 2 grams | **Keto Quarter Pounder**
• Fat: 34 grams
• 10 minutes of preparation
• Protein: 25 grams
• 8 minutes of cooking
• Net carbs: 4
• |
| Day 9 | **Easy Blender Pancakes**
• Fat: 29 grams
• 5 | **Broccoli Bacon Salad**
• Fat: 31 grams
• 15 minutes of preparation
• Protein: 10 grams | **Sardine Stuffed Avocados**
• Fat: 29 grams
• 10 |

	minutes of preparation • Protein: 41 grams • 10 minutes of cooking • Net carbs: 4 grams	• 6 minutes of cooking • Net carbs: 5 grams	minutes to prepare • Protein: 27 grams • 0 minutes to cook • Net Carbs: 5 grams
Day 10	**California Chicken Omelet** • Fat 32 grams • 10 minutes to prepare • Protein 25 grams • 10 minutes of cooking • Net Carb: 3 grams	**Shrimp Scampi** • Fat: 21 grams • 5 minutes to prepare • Protein: 21 grams • 30 minutes of cooking • Net carbs: 4 grams	**Tuna Tartare** • Fat: 36 grams • 15 minutes to prepare • Protein: 41 grams • 15 minutes of cooking • Net carbs: 4 grams
YOU DID IT!!	Congratulations! You have successfully completed a 10 day ketogenic cleanse. By now your body has adjusted to its new source of energy, expelled dozens of harmful toxins, and replenished itself with many vitamins and minerals it may have been lacking. Way		

	to go on a job well done!

CHAPTER 3: BREAKFAST IS FOR CHAMPIONS

Breakfast is by far the most important meal of the day for one reason: it set the tone for the rest of your day. In order to hit the ground running, it is vital that one starts each day with foods that fuel an energetic and productive day. This chapter contains ten ketogenic breakfast ideas that will have you burning fat and conquering your day like you never imagined.

1. CALIFORNIA CHICKEN OMELET

- This recipe requires 10 minutes of preparation, 10 minutes of cooking time and serves 1
- Net carbs: 4 grams
- Protein: 25 grams
- Fat : 32 grams

What you will need:

- Mayo (1 tablespoon)
- Mustard (1 teaspoon)
- Campari tomato
- Eggs (2 large beaten)
- Avocado (one-fourth, sliced)
- Bacon (2 slices cooked and chopped)
- Deli chicken (1 ounce)

What to do:

1. Place a skillet on the stove over a burner set to a medium heat and let it warm before adding the eggs and seasoning as needed.

2. Once eggs are cooked about halfway through, add bacon, chicken, avocado, tomato, mayo, and mustard on one side of the eggs.

3. Fold the omelet onto its self, cover and cook for 5 additional minutes.

4. Once eggs are fully cooked, and all ingredients are warm, through the center, your omelet is ready.

5. Bon apatite!

2. STEAK AND EGGS WITH AVOCADO

- This recipe requires 10 minutes of preparation, 5 minutes of cooking time and serves 1

- Net Carbs: 3 grams

- Protein: 44 grams

- Fat: 36 grams

What you will need:

- Salt and pepper

- Avocado (one-fourth, sliced)

- Sirloin steak (4 ounces)

- Eggs (3 large)

- Butter (1 tablespoon)

What to do:

1. Melt the tablespoon of butter in a pan and fry all 3 eggs to the desired doneness. Season the eggs with salt and pepper.

2. In a different pan, cook the sirloin steak to your preferred taste and slice it into thin strips. Season the steak with salt and pepper.

3. Sever your prepared steak and eggs with slices of avocado.

4. Enjoy!

3. PANCAKES IN A BLENDER

- This recipe requires 5 minutes of preparation, 10 minutes of cooking time and serves 1
- Net Carbs: 4 grams
- Protein: 41 grams
- Fat: 29 grams

What you will need:

- Whey protein powder (1 scoop)

- Eggs (2 large)

- Cream cheese (2 ounces)

- Just a pinch of cinnamon and a pinch of salt

What to do:

1. Combine cream cheese, eggs, protein powder, cinnamon, and salt in a blender. Blend for 10 seconds and let stand.

2. While letting batter stand, warm a skillet over medium heat.

3. Pour about ¼ of the batter into warmed skillet and let cook. When bubbles begin to emerge on the surface, flip the pancake.

4. Once flipped, cook for 15 seconds. Repeat until the remainder of the batter is used up.

5. Top with butter and/ or sugar- free maple syrup and you are all set!

6. Chow time!

4. LOW CARB SMOOTHE BOWL

- Net Carbs: 4 grams

- Protein: 35 grams

- Fat: 35 grams

- It takes 5 minutes to prepare and serves 1.

What you will need:

- Spinach (1 cup)

- Almond milk (half a cup)

- Coconut oil (1 tablespoon)

- Low carb protein powder (1 scoop)

- Ice cubes (2 cubes)

- Whipping cream (2 T)

- Optional toppings can include: raspberries, walnuts, shredded coconut, or chia seeds

What to do:

1. Place spinach in the blender. Add almond milk, cream, coconut oil, and ice. Blend until thoroughly and evenly combined.

2. Pour into bowl.

3. Top with toppings or stir lightly into a smoothie.

4. Treat yourself!

5. FETA AND PESTO OMELET

- This recipe requires 5 minutes of preparation, 5 minutes of cooking time and serves 1

- Net Carbs: 2.5 grams

- Protein: 30 grams

- Fat: 46 grams

What you will need:

- Butter (1 tablespoon)

- Eggs (3 large)

- Heavy cream (1 tablespoon)

- Feta cheese (1 ounce)

- Basil pesto (1 teaspoon)

- Tomatoes (optional)

What to do:

1. Heat pan and melt butter.

2. Beat eggs together with heavy whipping cream (will give eggs a fluffy consistency once cooked).

3. Pour eggs into pan and cook until almost done, add feta and pesto to on half of the eggs.

4. Fold omelet and cook for an additional 4-5 minutes.

5. Top with feta and tomatoes, and eat up!

6. CREPES WITH CREAM AND RASPBERRIES

- This recipe requires 5 minutes of preparation, 15 minutes of cooking time and serves 2

- Net Carbs: 8 grams

- Protein: 15 grams

- Fat: 40 grams

What you will need:

- Raspberries (3 ounces, fresh or frozen)

- Whole Milk Ricotta (half a cup and 2 tablespoons)

- Erythritol (2 tablespoons)

- Eggs (2 large)

- Cream Cheese (2 ounces)

- Pinch of salt

- Dash of Cinnamon

- Whipped cream and sugar- free maple syrup to go on top

What to do:

1. In a blender, blend cream cheese, eggs, erythritol, salt, and cinnamon for about 20 seconds, or until there are no lumps of cream cheese.

2. Place a pan on a burner turned to a medium heat before coating in cooking spray. Add 20 percent of your batter to the pan in a thin layer. Cook crepe until the underside becomes slightly darkened. Carefully flip the crepe and let the reverse side cook for about 15 seconds.

3. Repeat step 3 until all batter is used.

4. Without stacking the crepes, allow them to cool for a few minutes.

5. After the crepes have cool, place about 2 tablespoons of ricotta cheese in the center of each crepe.

6. Throw in a couple of raspberries and fold the side to the middle.

7. Top those off with some whipped cream and sugar- free maple syrup and...

8. Viola! You're a true chef! Indulge in your creation!

7. GREEN MONSTER SMOOTHIE

- This recipe requires 10 minutes of preparation, 0 minutes of cooking time and serves 1
- Net Carbs: 4 grams
- Protein: 30 grams
- Fat: 25 grams

What you will need:

- Almond milk (one and a half cups)
- Spinach (one-eighth of a cup)
- Cucumber (a fourth of a cup)
- Celery (a fourth of a cup)
- Avocado (a fourth of a cup)
- Coconut oil (1 tablespoon)
- Stevia (liquid, 10 drops)
- Whey Protein Powder (1 scoop)

What to do:

1. In a blender, blend almond milk and spinach for a few pulses.

2. Add remaining ingredients and blend until thoroughly combined.

3. Add optional matcha powder, if desired, and enjoy!

CHAPTER 4: LUNCH CRUNCH

Eating a healthy lunch when you are limited on time due to, work, school, or taking care of your kids can be a tumultuous task. Thankfully, we have compiled a list of eight quick and easy recipes to accompany the ten-day meal plan laid out in chapter 2! Many find it advantageous, especially if you work throughout the week, to prepare your meals ahead of time. Thankfully, these lunch recipes are also easy to pack and take on the go!

1. OFF THE COBB SALAD

- Net carbs: 3 grams
- Protein: 43 grams
- Fat: 48 grams
- It takes 10 minutes to prepare and serves 1.

What you will need:

- Spinach (1 cup)
- Egg (1, hard-boiled)
- Bacon (2 strips)
- Chicken breast (2 ounces)
- Campari tomato (one-half of tomato)
- Avocado (one-fourth, sliced)
- White vinegar (half of a teaspoon)
- Olive oil (1 tablespoon)

What to do:

1. Cook chicken and bacon completely and cut or slice into small pieces.
2. Chop remaining ingredients into bite size pieces.
3. Place all ingredients, including chicken and bacon, in a bowl, toss ingredients in oil and vinegar.
4. Enjoy!

2. AVOCADO AND SARDINES

- Net Carbs: 5 grams

- Protein: 27 grams

- Fat: 52 grams

- It takes 10 minutes to prepare and serves 1.

What you will need:

- Fresh lemon juice (1 tablespoon)

- Spring onion or chives (1 or small bunch)

- Mayonnaise (1 tablespoon)

- Sardines (1 tin, drained)

- Avocado (1 whole, seed removed)

- Turmeric powder (a fourth of a teaspoon) or freshly ground turmeric root (1 teaspoon)

- Salt (a fourth of a teaspoon)

What to do:

1. Begin by cutting the avocado in half and removing its seed.

2. Scoop out about half the avocado and set aside (shown below).

3. In a small bowl, mash drained sardines with a fork.

4. Add onion (or chives), turmeric powder, and mayonnaise. Mix well.

5. Add removed avocado to sardine mixture.

6. Add lemon juice and salt.

7. Scoop the mixture into avocado halves.

8. Dig in!

3. CHICKEN SALAD A LA PESTO

- This recipe requires 5minutes of preparation, 10 minutes of cooking time and serves 4
- Net Carbs: 3 grams
- Protein: 27 grams
- Fat: 27 grams

What you will need:

- Garlic pesto (2 tablespoons)
- Mayonnaise (a fourth of a cup)
- Grape tomatoes (10, halved)
- Avocado (1, cubed)
- Bacon (6 slices, cooked crisp and crumbled)
- Chicken (1 pound, cooked and cubed)
- Romaine lettuce (optional)

What to do:

1. Combine all ingredients in a large mixing bowl.

2. Toss gently to spread mayonnaise and pesto evenly throughout.

3. If desired, wrap in romaine lettuce for a low-carb BLT chicken wrap.

4. Bon apatite!

4. BACON AND ROASTED BRUSSEL SPROUTS

- This recipe requires 5 minutes of preparation, 30 minutes of cooking time and serves 4
- Net Carbs: 4 grams
- Protein: 15 grams
- Fat: 21 grams

What you will need:

- Bacon (8 strips)
- Olive oil (2 tablespoons)
- Brussel sprouts (1 pound, halved)
- Salt and pepper

What to do:

1. Preheat oven to 375 degrees Fahrenheit.
2. Gently mix Brussel sprouts with olive oil, salt, and pepper.
3. Spread Brussel sprouts evenly onto a greased baking sheet.

4. Bake in the oven for 30 minutes. Shake the pan about halfway through to mix the Brussel sprout halves up a bit.

5. While Brussel sprouts are in the oven, fry bacon slices on the stovetop.

6. When bacon is fully cooked, let cool and chop it into bite size pieces.

7. Combine Bacon and Brussel sprouts in a bowl, and you're finished!

8. Feast!!

5. GRILLED HALLOUMI SALAD

- Net Carbs: 7 grams

- Protein: 21 grams

- Fat: 47 grams

- It takes 15 minutes to prepare and serves 1.

What you will need:

- Chopped walnuts (half of an ounce)

- Baby arugula (1 handful)

- Grape tomatoes (5)

- Cucumber (1)

- Halloumi cheese (3 ounces)

- Olive oil (1 teaspoon)

- Balsamic vinegar (half of a teaspoon)

- A pinch of salt

What to do:

1. Slice halloumi cheese into slices 1/3 of an in thick.

2. Grill cheese for 3 to 5 minutes, until you see grill lines, on each side.

3. Wash and cut veggies into bite size pieces, place in salad bowl.

4. Add rinsed baby arugula and walnuts to veggies.

5. Toss in olive oil, balsamic vinegar, and salt.

6. Place grilled halloumi on top of veggies, and your lunch is ready!

7. Eat those greens and get back to work!

6. BACON BROCCOLI SALAD

- This recipe requires 15 minutes of preparation, 6 minutes of cooking time and serves 5.
- Net Carbs: 5 grams
- Protein: 10 grams
- Fat: 31 grams

What you will need:

- Sesame oil (half of a teaspoon)
- Erythritol (1 and a half tablespoons) or stevia to taste
- White vinegar (1 tablespoon)
- Mayonnaise (half of a cup)
- Green onion (three-fourths of an ounce)
- Bacon (a fourth of a pound)
- Broccoli (1 pound, heads, and stalks cut and trimmed)

What to do:

1. Cook bacon and crumble into bits.

2. Cut broccoli into bite sized pieces.

3. Slice scallions.

4. Mix mayonnaise, vinegar, erythritol (or stevia), and sesame oil, to make the dressing.

5. Place broccoli and bacon bits in a bowl and toss with dressing.

6. Viola!

7. TUNA AVOCADO TARTARE

- Net Carbs: 4 grams

- Protein: 56 grams

- Fat: 24 grams

- It takes 15 minutes to prepare and serves 2.

What you will need:

- Sesame seed oil (2 tablespoons)

- Sesame seeds (1 teaspoon)

- Cucumbers (2)

- Lime (half of a whole lime)

- Mayonnaise (1 tablespoon)

- Sriracha (1 tablespoon)

- Olive oil (2 tablespoons)

- Jalapeno (one-half of the whole jalapeno)

- Scallion (3 stalks)

- Avocado (1)

- Tuna steak (1 pound)

\- Soy sauce (1 tablespoon)

What to do:

1. Dice tuna and avocado into ¼ inch cubes, place in a bowl.

2. Finely chop scallion and jalapeno, add to bowl.

3. Pour olive oil, sesame oil, sriracha, soy sauce, mayonnaise, and lime into a bowl.

4. Using hands, toss all ingredients to combine evenly. Using a utensil may breakdown avocado, which you want to remain chunky, so it is best to use your hands.

5. Top with sesame seeds and serve with a side of sliced cucumber.

6. There's certainly something fishy about this recipe, but it tastes great! Enjoy!

8. WARM SPINACH AND SHRIMP

- This recipe requires 15 minutes of preparation, 6 minutes of cooking time and serves 5.
- Fat: 24 grams
- Protein: 36 grams
- Net Carbs: 3 grams
- Takes10 minutes to prepare, 5 minutes to cook, and serves 2.

What you will need:

- Spinach (2 handfuls)
- Parmesan (half a tablespoon)
- Heavy cream (1 tablespoon)
- Olive oil (1 tablespoon)
- Butter (2 tablespoons)
- Garlic (3 cloves)
- Onion (one fourth of whole onion)

- Large raw shrimp (about 20)

- Lemon (optional)

What to do:

1. Place peeled shrimp in cold water.

2. Chop onions and garlic into fine pieces.

3. Heat oil in a pan, over medium heat. Cook shrimp in oil until lightly pink (we do not want them fully cooked here). Remove shrimp from oil and set aside.

4. Place chopped onions and garlic into the pan, cook until onions are translucent. Add a dash of salt.

5. Add butter, cream, and parmesan cheese. Stir until you have a smooth sauce.

6. Let the sauce cook for about 2 minutes, so it will thicken slightly.

7. Place shrimp back into the pan and cook until done. This should take no longer than 2 or 3

minutes. Be careful not to overcook the shrimp; it will become dry and tough!

8. Remove shrimp and sauce from pan and replace with spinach. Cook spinach VERY briefly

9. Place warmed spinach onto a plate.

10. Pour shrimp and sauce over a bed of spinach, squeeze some lemon on top, if you like, and you're ready to chow down!

CHAPTER 5: THINNER BY DINNER

It's the end of the day and you are winding down from a hard day's work. Your body does not require a lot of energy while you sleep; therefore, dinner will typically consist of less fat and more protein.

1. CHICKEN PAD THAI

- Net Carbs: 7 grams

- Protein: 30 grams

- Fat: 12 grams

- It takes 15 minutes to prepare, 15 minutes to cook, and serves 4.

What you will need:

- Peanuts (1 ounce)

- Lime (1 whole)

- Soy sauce (2 tablespoons)

- Egg (1 large)

- Zucchini (2 large)

- Chicken thighs (16 ounces, boneless and skinless)
- Garlic (2 cloves, minced)
- White onion (1,chopped)
- Olive oil (1 tablespoon)
- Chili flakes (optional)

What to do:

1. Over medium heat, cook olive oil and onion until translucent. Add the garlic and cook about three minutes (until fragrant).
2. Cook chicken in the pan for 5 to 7 minutes on each side (until fully cooked). Remove chicken from heat and shred it using a couple of forks.
3. Cut ends off zucchini and cut into thin noodles. Set zucchini noodles aside.
4. Next, scramble the egg in the pan.
5. Once the egg is fully cooked, and the zucchini noodles and cook for about 2 minutes.

6. Add the previously shredded chicken to the pan.

7. Give it some zing with soy sauce, lime juice, peanuts, and chili flakes.

8. Time to eat!

2. CHIPOTLE STYLE FISH TACOS

- Fat: 20 grams

- Protein: 24 grams

- Net Carbs: 7 grams

- It takes 5 minutes to prepare, 15 minutes to cook, and serves 4.

What you will need:

- Low carb tortillas (4)

- Haddock fillets (1 pound)

- Mayonnaise (2 tablespoons)

- Butter (2 tablespoons)

- Chipotle peppers in adobo sauce (4 ounces)

- Garlic (2 cloves, pressed)

- Jalapeño (1 fresh, chopped)

- Olive oil (2 tablespoons)

- Yellow onion (half of an onion, diced)

What to do:

1. Fry diced onion (until translucent) in olive oil in a high sided pan, over medium- high heat.

2. Reduce heat to medium, add jalapeno and garlic. Cook while stirring for another two minutes.

3. Chop the chipotle peppers and add them, along with the adobo sauce, to the pan.

4. Add the butter, mayo, and fish fillets to the pan.

5. Cook the fish fully while breaking up the fillets and stirring the fish into other ingredients.

6. Warm tortillas for 2 minutes on each side.

7. Fill tortillas with fishy goodness and eat up!

3. SALMON WITH AVOCADO LIME SAUCE

- Net Carbs: 5 grams

- Protein: 37 grams

- Fat: 27 grams

- It takes 20 minutes to prepare, 10 minutes to cook, and serves 2.

What you will need:

- Salmon (two 6 ounce fillets)
- Avocado (1 large)
- Lime (one-half of a whole lime)
- Red onion (2 tablespoons, diced)
- Cauliflower (100 grams)

What to do:

1. Chop cauliflower in a blender or food processor then cooks it in a lightly oiled pan,

while covered, for 8 minutes. This will make the cauliflower rice-like.

2. Next, blend the avocado with squeezed lime juice in the blender or processor until smooth and creamy.

3. Heat some oil in a skillet and cook salmon (skin side down first) for 4 to 5 minute. Flip the fillets and cook for an additional 4 to 5 minutes.

4. Place salmon fillet on a bed of your cauliflower rice and top with some diced red onion.

4. SIRACHA LIME STEAK

- Net Carbs: 5 grams

- Protein: 48 grams

- Fat: 32 grams

- It takes 5 minutes to prepare, 10 minutes to cook, and serves 2.

What you will need:

- Vinegar (1 teaspoon)

- Olive oil (2 tablespoons)

- Lime (1 whole)

- Sriracha (2 tablespoons)

- Flank steak (16 ounces)

- Salt and pepper

What to do:

1. Season steak, liberally, with salt and pepper. Place on baking sheet, lined with foil, and broil in oven for 5 minutes on each side (add

another minute or two for a well-done steak). Remove from oven, cover, and set aside.

2. Place sriracha in a small bowl and squeeze lime into it. Whisk in salt, pepper, and vinegar.

3. Slowly pour in olive oil.

4. Slice steak into thin slices, slather on your sauce, and enjoy!

5. Feel free to pair this recipe with a side of greens such as asparagus or broccoli.

5. LOW CARB SESAME CHICKEN

- Net Carbs: 4 grams
- Protein: 45 grams
- Fat: 36 grams
- Takes 15minutes to prepare, 15 minutes to cook, and serves 2.

What you will need:

- Broccoli (three-fourths of a cup, cut bite size)
- Xanthan gum (a fourth of a teaspoon)

- Sesame seeds (2 tablespoons)

- Garlic (1 clove)

- Ginger (1 cm cube)

- Vinegar (1 tablespoon)

- Brown sugar alternative (Sukrin Gold is a good one) (2 tablespoons)

- Soy sauce (2 tablespoons)

- Toasted sesame seed oil (2 tablespoons)

- Arrowroot powder or cornstarch (1 tablespoon)

- Chicken thighs (1poundcut into bite sized pieces)

- Egg (1 large)

- Salt and pepper

- Chives (optional)

What to do:

1. First, we will make the batter by combining the egg with a tablespoon of arrowroot powder (or cornstarch). Whisk well.

2. Place chicken pieces in batter. Be sure to coat all sides of chicken pieces with the batter.

3. Heat one tablespoon of sesame oil, in a large pan. Add chicken pieces to hot oil and fry. Be gentle when flipping the chicken, you want to keep the batter from falling off. It should take about 10 minutes for them to cook fully.

4. Next, make the sesame sauce. In a small bowl, combine soy sauce, brown sugar alternative, vinegar, ginger, garlic, sesame seeds, and the remaining tablespoon of toasted sesame seed oil. Whisk very well.

5. Once the chicken is fully cooked, add broccoli and the sesame sauce to the pan and cook for an additional 5 minutes.

6. Spoon desired amount into a bowl, top it off with some chopped chives, and relish in some fine dining at home!

6. PAN 'O SAUSAGE

- Net Carbs: 4 grams

- Protein: 30 grams

- Fat: 38 grams

- It takes 10 minutes to prepare, 25 minutes to cook, and serves 2.

What you will need:

- Basil (half a teaspoon)

- Oregano (half a teaspoon)

- White onion (1 tablespoon)

- Shredded mozzarella (a fourth of a cup)

- Parmesan cheese (a fourth of a cup)

- Vodka sauce (half a cup)

- Mushrooms (4 ounces)

- Sausage (3 links)

- Salt (a fourth of a teaspoon)

- Red pepper (a fourth of a teaspoon, ground)

What to do:

1. Preheat oven to 350 degrees Fahrenheit.

2. Heat an iron skillet over medium flame. When skillet is hot, cook sausage links until almost thoroughly cooked.

3. While sausage is cooking, slice mushrooms and onion.

4. When sausage is almost fully cooked, remove links from heat and place mushrooms and onions in skillet until brown.

5. Cut sausage into pieces about ½ inch thick and place pieces in the pan.

6. Season skillet contents with oregano, basil, salt, and red pepper.

7. Add vodka sauce and parmesan cheese. Stir everything together.

8. Place skillet in oven for 15 minutes. Sprinkle mozzarella on top a couple minutes before removing the dish from oven.

9. Once 15 minutes is up, remove skillet from the oven and let cool for a few minutes.

10. Dinner time!

7. QUARTER POUNDER KETO BURGER

- Net Carbs: 4 grams

- Protein: 25 grams

- Fat: 34 grams

- Takes 10 minutes to prepare, 8 minutes to cook, and serves 2.

What you will need:

- Basil (half a teaspoon)

- Cayenne (fourth a teaspoon)

- Crushed red pepper (half a teaspoon)

- Salt (half a teaspoon)

- Lettuce (2 large leaves)

- Butter (2 tablespoons)

- Egg (1 large)

- Sriracha (1 tablespoon)

- Onion (fourth of whole onion)

- Plum tomato (half of the whole tomato)

- Mayo (1 tablespoon)

- Pickled jalapenos (1 tablespoon, sliced)

- Bacon (1 strip)

- Ground beef (half a pound)

- Bacon (1 strip)

What to do:

1. Knead mean for about three minutes.

2. Chop bacon, jalapeno, tomato, and onion into fine pieces. (shown below)

3. Knead in mayo, sriracha, egg, and chopped ingredients, and spices into the meat.

4. Separate meat into four even pieces and flatten them (not thinly, just press on the tops to create a flat surface). Place a tablespoon of butter on top of two of the meat pieces. Take the pieces that do not have butter in them and set them on top of the buttered ones (basically

creating a butter and meat sandwich). Seal the sides together, concealing the butter within.

5. Throw the patties on the grill (or in a pan) for about 5 minutes on each side. Caramelize some onions if you want too!

6. Prepare large leaves of lettuce by spreading some mayo onto them. Once patties are finished, place them on one-half of the lettuce, add your desired burger toppings, and fold the other half over of the lettuce leaf over the patty.

7. Burger time!

About The Author

Hi there it's Diana here, I want to share a little bit about myself so that we can get to know each other on a deeper level. I grew up in California and have lived there for the better part of my life. Being exposed to many different cultures, people, and food, those experiences have certainly influenced my style of cooking and shaped my perception of the world in many profound ways. Cooking has always been a passion of mine since I was young and I made it a goal to one day become a master chef, bringing food to people that are one-of-a-kind. Fast forward a few decades and I have succeeded in my dreams which I am extremely grateful and proud of. With my husband and two kids, I now live a very happy and fulfilled life. One I wouldn't trade anything in the world for.

www.ingramcontent.com/pod-product-compliance
Lightning Source LLC
LaVergne TN
LVHW011113181125
825886LV00009B/254